THE BAKING SODA
SECRET

HOW TO REVIVE YOUR LIFE WITH THIS
SIMPLE KITCHEN CABINET MIRACLE

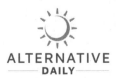

ALTERNATIVE
DAILY

This page intentionally left blank.

This page intentionally left blank.

Table of Contents

Introduction 13

The History of Baking Soda & What It Is 14

   The Roots of Baking Soda in its Current Form............................ 15

   Baking Soda: Mid-19th Century to Today 16

   The Difference Between Baking Soda and Baking Powder.................. 17

Baking Soda Fun Facts... 19

   Baking Soda Has Its Own Day 20

   The Chemical Formula and Where It's Mined............................ 20

   It Has A Lot of Names.. 21

   Baking Soda Isn't the Same as Baking Powder........................... 22

   You Can Make Glow Worms With It 23

   You Can Make Invisible Ink With It 24

   You Can Use It As a Toothpaste and a Mouthwash....................... 25

   It Will Kill Roaches 26

   A Fun Party Trick.. 27

   Baking Soda Can Reduce CO2 in our Planet's Atmosphere.................. 28

How Baking Soda Can Help Protect the Environment............... 30

Replacing Standard Household Cleaners with Baking Soda 31

Replacing Personal Care Products with Baking Soda 34

Pets and Baking Soda **36**

Cleaning Products, Shampoos, Flea Repellents and Beyond 37

Countless Unnecessary Deaths Related to Insect Repellant Products 39

How Baking Soda Can Help 39

Ways to Use Baking Soda as a Healthier, Effective Alternative 40

Killing Fleas 40

Eliminating Odors 43

Clean Up an Accident 44

Clean and Deodorize Bedding 44

Remove that Awful Skunk Smell 45

Give Fido a Dry Bath 46

Clean Dog Toys 46

Clean Food and Water Bowls 47

Relieve the Pain of a Bee Sting 47

Gardening and Baking Soda **48**

An Alternative Pesticide 51

Revive Lifeless Plants 53

Get Rid of Weeds and Crabgrass 53

Test the pH of Your Garden Soil 54

Treat Tomato Diseases 56

Grow Sweeter Tomatoes 56

Deodorize Your Compost Bin or Pile 57

Clean Garden and Patio Furniture 57

Cooking with Baking Soda: Tips and Tricks **58**

Brown Onions Faster 59

Get Crispier Chicken 59

Counteract a Too-Strong Vinegar Taste 60

Bake Beans That Minimize Gas Production.. 60

Make Softer Beans to Use in Hummus.. 61

Make Fluffier Omelets.. 62

Lighter, Softer Waffles... 62

Tenderize Meat and Poultry 62

Reduce the Acidity of Tomatoes.. 63

Transform Angel Hair Pasta Into Ramen Noodles............................. 64

Clarify Iced Tea 66

Clean Up Your Produce 66

Reduce a Fishy Taste.. 67

Preparing a Fresh, Whole Chicken 67

Soften the Pungent Taste of Wild Game 67

Improve the Texture of Shrimp 68

Neutralize the Acids in a Fruit Recipe 68

Reduce Acidity in Common Beverages 69

Make Chocolate Cake Darker 69

Prevent Homemade Frosting From Cracking 70

Stop Milk From Curdling When Boiling... 70

Get Fluffier Rice 70

Cleaning With Baking Soda **71**

The Dangers of the Chemicals in Traditional Cleaning Supplies 72

Baking Soda: A Better Alternative.. 74

Your Entire Home **75**

All-Purpose Cleaner 75

Air Freshener.. 77

Your Kitchen **79**

Produce Cleaner 79

Oven Cleaner 80

A Drain Cleaner... 83

Floor Cleaner.. 84

Scour a Ceramic Cooktop... 85

Renew Burned Stainless Steel Cookware.. 85

Make Your Silver Sparkle Again.. 86

Dishwasher Cleaner 86

Refrigerator Cleaner 86

Refreshing Stale-Smelling Sponges... 87

Living Room.. **88**

Carpet Freshener.. 88

Deodorize Musty Upholstery 88

Remove Grime From Your Couch.. 88

Removing Water Stains From Wood Coffee Tables............................ 89

Bathrooms **90**

    Toilet Bowl Cleaner 90

    Shower and Tub Cleaner 91

    Glass Shower Doors 91

    Drains and Faucets 92

    Hair Brush Cleaner 93

    Toothbrush Cleaner 93

    Deodorizing a Front-Load Washer 94

    Keep Linen Closet Odors Away 94

Outdoor Areas **95**

    Cleaning Dirty Patio Furniture 95

    Get Rid of Garbage Can Odors 95

    Clean Up the BBQ Grill 95

Baking Soda For Your Health **96**

    Get Rid of Ingrown Hairs 97

    A Homemade Deodorant 98

    Flu-Proof Frequently Touched Surfaces in Your Room 99

    Sanitize Cutting Boards 99

    Control Burping 100

    Relieve Acid Reflux and Heartburn Pain 100

    Halt a Mosquito Bite Itch in its Tracks 101

    Relieve Sensitive Teeth 101

    Reduce Inflammation 102

Treat Swollen Feet...102

Prevent Foot Odor and Microbial Infections 103

A Foot Exfoliator...104

Soothe Chafing 105

Eczema Relief 106

Ease Cold and Flu Symptoms..108

Balance pH to Promote Better Health...109

Relieve the Discomfort of a Urinary Tract Infection 109

Possible Cancer Prevention and Support For Those With Cancer.......110

Preventing and Relieving Painful Kidney Stones 111

Treating Kidney Disease 112

Reduce the Risk of Osteoporosis 113

Enhance Workouts..114

Treating Hyperkalemia..115

Decreasing the Pain and Swelling of a Bee or Wasp Sting 116

Minimize Metabolic Acidosis...116

Baking Soda For Beauty **117**

Deodorant 121

Toothpaste and Whitener 122

Mouthwash 123

Shampoo...124

Dry Shampoo...125

Get Rid of Chlorine Hair 126

Wash Dreadlocks..127

Acne Mask 128

Beautify Your Feet..129

Keep Your Combs and Brushes Clean 131

Gently Cleaning Extra-Dirty Hands 132

Enhance a Manicure 133

Brighten Your Complexion..134

Heal a Rash..135

Artificial Tan Remover 136

Soothe Razor Burn..137

Relieve Itchy Skin..138

Exfoliate Your Face For a Beautiful, Glowing Look 139

Fade Dark Spots, Moles and Freckles.............................140

Soothe a Sunburn 142

Remove Facial Hair 143

Stock Up **144**

This page intentionally left blank.

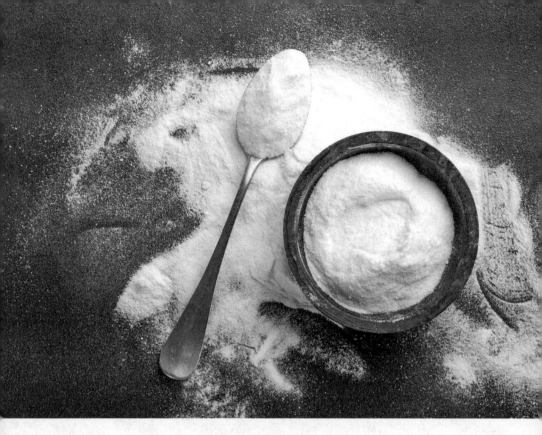

Introduction

Welcome to the wonderful world of baking soda. Who would have thought that such a simple and natural substance could do so much! You will be amazed at the versatility of this white powder. It's capable of tackling the most potent cleaning jobs while still being soft enough to use as an ingredient for your favorite face wash or tooth powder. Baking soda is not just for baking! It has so many applications for your house, health, garden and even your pets.

We have put together the best information available on baking soda and it is our hope that this book will serve you as a great reference for many years to come!

Enjoy!

The History of Baking Soda & What It Is

Baking soda is 100 percent bicarbonate of soda. It's alkaline in nature and creates carbon dioxide bubbles when it's combined with an acid, giving rise to dough and batters — it acts as a leavening agent. Common acids used to cause the reaction including vinegar, cream of tartar, yogurt, buttermilk and lemon juice.

Although many people get it mixed up with baking powder, the two are not the same, and neither are they interchangeable in recipes. The natural mineral form of baking soda is called nahcolite, which is a component of the mineral natron that can be found in many springs.

Sodium bicarbonate has a rich history, which extends thousands of years into our past. Ancient Egyptians used natural deposits of the mineral natron as paint for their hieroglyphics. They also used the substance for treating wounds, cleaning the teeth and gums, drying and preserving meats, removing oil and grease, and to help preserve the dead as mummies.

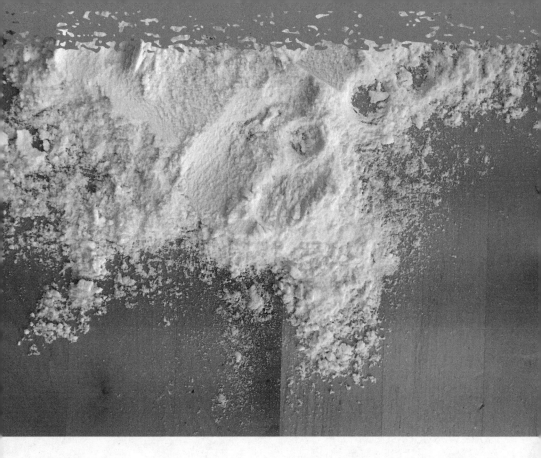

The Roots of Baking Soda in its Current Form

The root of baking soda in its current form dates back to 1791, when French chemist Nicholas Leblanc produced sodium carbonate, or soda ash. It was in the mid-19th century that two New York bakers, John Dwight and his brother-in-law Austin Church, opened up the first U.S. factory designed to produce baking soda from carbon dioxide and sodium carbonate as a leavening agent for baked goods. In fact, that's where Arm & Hammer, the famous company that sells baking soda in the little orange box, got its start. Church & Company was formed to meet the increasing demand for baking soda, and the Arm & Hammer trademark, showing the arm of Vulcan (the Roman god of fire) bringing down his hammer on an anvil, was meant to symbolize its strength.

Baking Soda: Mid-19th Century to Today

Saleratus, or sodium carbonate, was mentioned in the novel "Captains Courageous" by Rudyard Kipling as being used extensively in the 1800s for commercial fishing in order to prevent freshly caught fish from spoiling. As it became readily available, sodium bicarbonate was found to be useful in a myriad of applications. In the late 1920s, national magazines such as *McCall's* and *Good Housekeeping* started promoting its usefulness in the home. The first full-color ad for baking soda was published in the 1960s.

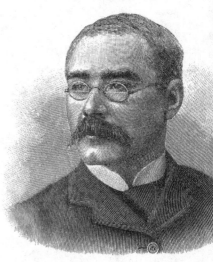

Rudyard Kipling.

In 1970, when Arm & Hammer became the sole sponsor of the first annual Earth Day, baking soda gained attention around the world as the "go-to" eco-friendly alternative to chemical cleaners. And, in 1972, a new use for baking soda received widespread attention. The word got out about Americans using it in their refrigerators to keep food fresh and odors out. By the mid-1980s, it had gotten so popular that as part of its 100th birthday celebration, the inner copper walls of the Statue of Liberty were cleaned and restored using baking soda, which removed 99 years of grime.

Today, baking soda is even included in the World Health Organization's list of essential medicines. A 2002 United Nations Environment Programme (UNEP) publication reported that the majority of sodium bicarbonate global applications were for food uses, and about 5% in cosmetics.

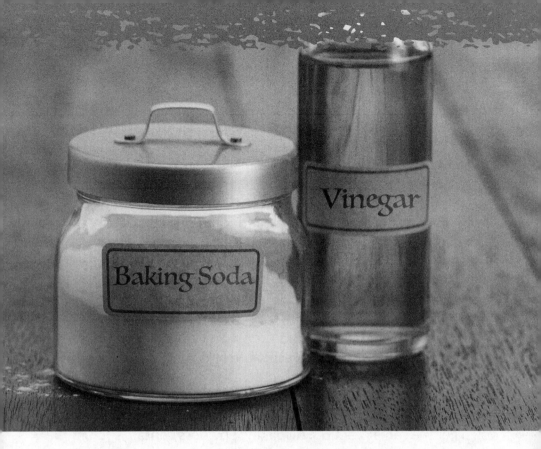

The Difference Between Baking Soda and Baking Powder

Some people are confused as to whether or not baking soda can be substituted for baking powder, or vice versa, in cooking, with the belief that they're basically one in the same. While baking soda and baking powder are both leaveners used in baking, they are chemically different and cannot be used interchangeably.

The easiest way to explain the differences is to start with the knowledge that baking soda is an alkaline base. Do you recall those experiments you did as a kid? Things like adding vinegar to baking soda to create a volcano eruption?

When you mix a base like baking soda with an acid like vinegar, you'll get a reaction, meaning that it will bubble up, or foam. In a baking recipe that requires baking soda, typically that recipe will have some kind of acid element, like vinegar, yogurt, lemon juice or buttermilk. When the two come together, carbon dioxide bubbles are formed, which creates the leavening in batter or dough. Baking soda creates leavening on its own when heated. You can try it as an experiment: Pour some boiling water over baking soda in a sink and watch what happens. If baking soda isn't balanced by adding an acidic ingredient, the taste is likely to be metallic.

Baking powder, on the other hand, is made up of a number of elements, including sodium bicarbonate or baking soda. It also includes an acid, cream of tartar and a filler, such as corn flour, which serves to absorb moisture. As it already has an acid in it, it doesn't need to be combined with acid, all you need to do is add water and you'll get the same reaction. All baking powders contain sodium bicarbonate, but baking powder also contains two acids, including monocalcium phosphate. Monocalcium phosphate doesn't react with sodium bicarbonate while it's dry, but as soon as the baking powder is stirred into a wet dough or batter, the two begin to react, releasing bubbles of carbon dioxide, and causing chemical leavening.

Now does it all make sense?

Baking Soda Fun Facts

Sodium bicarbonate, better known as baking soda, is a chemical compound that's primarily used in cooking and baking as a leavening agent, to deodorize and as a very effective cleaning agent. But it has such a long list of uses, it's almost magical, despite being surprisingly simple, mined in its natural form — nahcolite — as a white or colorless carbonate mineral.

In fact, there are a lot of things you probably don't know about this substance.

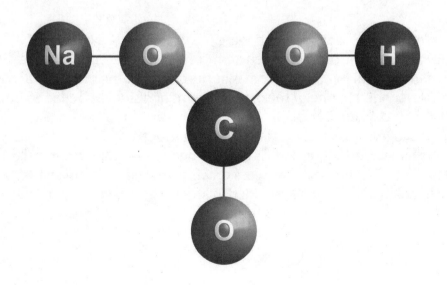

Baking Soda Has Its Own Day

That's right! December 30, the day before New Year's Eve, is actually National Bicarbonate of Soda Day. If you want to celebrate, try to use it in as many ways as you can come up with, or just build a baking soda and vinegar volcano and watch it explode.

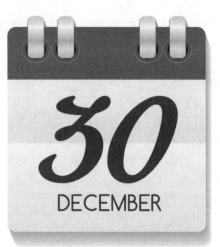

The Chemical Formula and Where It's Mined

The formula for sodium bicarbonate is CHNaO3. It's made up of one carbon atom, one hydrogen atom, one sodium atom and three oxygen atoms. The carbon atom is at the center of the molecule and is double-bonded to one of the oxygen atoms and single-bonded to the other two oxygen atoms. The oxygen atoms are, in turn, bonded to the hydrogen and sodium atoms, which are located on opposite sides of the molecule. Baking soda is alkaline and it has a molecular weight of 84.01. Nahcolite, that colorless or white mineral that consists of pure sodium bicarbonate, is mined in areas where lakes have dried up.

It Has A Lot of Names

As it's been known for so long and is so widely used, baking soda goes by many different names, in addition to sodium bicarbonate. Sometimes it's bicarbonate of soda, other times, cooking soda or even bread soda. There are other forms too, like bicarb soda, sodium bicarb or simply bicarb or bicarbonate. The word saleratus, from Latin *sal æratus* meaning "aerated salt," was commonly used in the 19th century for both sodium bicarbonate and potassium bicarbonate.

Baking Soda Isn't the Same as Baking Powder

Many people get baking soda and baking powder mixed up, but it can make a big difference depending on the purpose it's being used for. While baking powder is also sold for cooking and baking, it contains around 30% of HCO and various acidic ingredients that are activated by the addition of water, without requiring additional acids in the cooking medium. Many forms of baking powder do contain sodium bicarbonate, however, that's

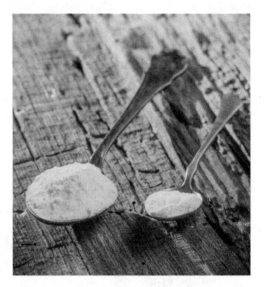

combined with calcium acid phosphate, sodium aluminium phosphate or cream of tartar. Baking soda is alkaline, while the acid used in baking powder avoids a metallic taste when the chemical change during baking creates sodium carbonate.

Baking soda is simply sodium bicarbonate with no other ingredient added. It's a base that reacts when it comes into contact with acids like vinegar or buttermilk. That reaction produces carbon dioxide in the form of bubbles like a liquid foam. Picture those school science experiments like fake volcanoes. When used for making baked goods, it makes the dough or batter rise due to a process called "chemical leavening."

You Can Make Glow Worms With It

One of the most fun things you can do with baking soda, other than those erupting volcanoes, is to make glow worms, also referred to as black snakes. All you need is that sodium bicarbonate, some alcohol, powdered sugar and sand.

To make it, combine four parts powdered sugar with one part baking soda. Make a mound with the sand and then create a depression in the middle using your thumbs. Pour alcohol over the mound to wet it, and then pour the baking soda/sugar mixture into the depression. Now, when you're ready, light it on fire and step back. First you'll see a little flame and a few black, scattered balls. When the reaction sets in, the carbon dioxide will puff up the baking soda into a "worm" or "snake" that continues to extrude while it smokes.

The whole thing occurs because the baking soda is breaking down into water vapor, sodium carbonate and carbon dioxide, and the sugar also has a reaction. It burns in oxygen, producing water vapor and carbon dioxide gas. Who knew that that little orange box in kitchens around the world could be so much fun? Forget about those pricey toys and high-tech gadgets, you can have fun with baking soda for hours with just a little knowledge.

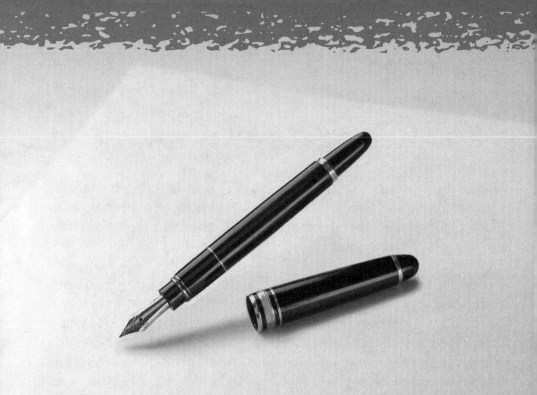

You Can Make Invisible Ink With It

Who hasn't thought about an invisibility superpower? While there still isn't away to make yourself invisible, you can harness its power to make invisible ink, which is still pretty cool. Just mix equal parts of water and baking soda to create your "ink." Now, dip a paintbrush, quill or toothpick into it and then draw or write onto a piece of paper. Let the paper dry completely. You can make the drawing or letters appear by either holding the paper close to a heat source like a lighter flame, stove or hot lightbulb, which causes a dark brown color, or pour grape juice over the paper and the invisible ink will become visible in a different hue.

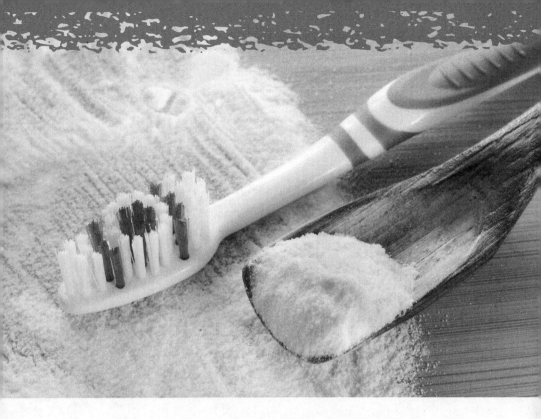

You Can Use It As a Toothpaste and a Mouthwash

You probably know that baking soda is an ingredient found in many toothpaste formulas. That's because it provides whitening properties in addition to removing plaque, thanks to its abrasive nature. You might find it in mouthwash too.

If you ever find yourself out of toothpaste, and you have a box of baking soda lying around, you can use that in a pinch, along with a little water, just enough to make a paste. It's a great toothpaste alternative; it acts as an antiseptic to neutralize the production of acids. By combining three parts of baking soda to one part water, you can use it to swish around in your mouth and eradicate even the most powerful smells, like garlic and onion.

It Will Kill Roaches

While roaches can seem nearly impossible to kill, sodium bicarbonate, combined with sugar, can do that trick without resorting to hazardous chemicals. The sweet smell of sugar will entice the roach to come out of its hiding place to eat. Simply mix together equal parts of baking soda and sugar in a small dish or something like a gallon milk jug lid. Set another small dish nearby and fill it with water. The roach will eat the sugar, along with the baking soda. When it heads to the water dish, the baking soda reacts. This creates gas inside of the roach, causing its stomach to burst.

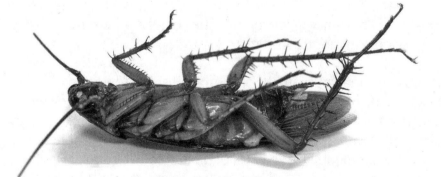

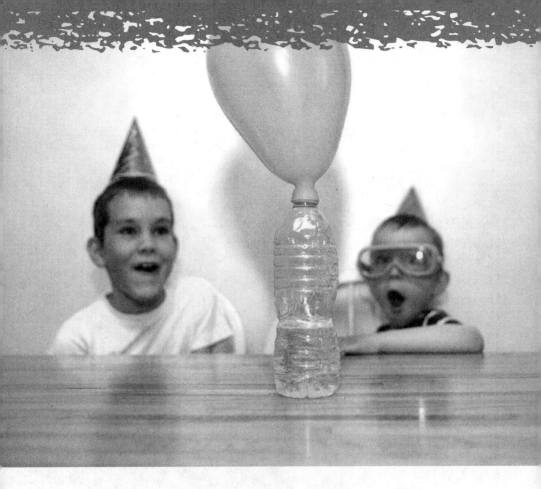

A Fun Party Trick

You can inflate a balloon using baking soda for an especially fun party trick. First, inflate a small balloon to stretch it out. Then, fill up the deflated balloon with two teaspoons of baking soda, using a small funnel to get it inside. Now, place four tablespoons of white vinegar into an empty plastic bottle. Place the end of the balloon over the bottle opening, tip the balloon up so that baking soda flows into the bottle and hold the end of the balloon in place. Watch what happens: the balloon will inflate, like magic!

Baking Soda Can Reduce CO2 in our Planet's Atmosphere

Scientists from the Lawrence Livermore National Laboratory in collaboration with researchers from the University of Illinois at Urbana-Champaign and Harvard University may have stumbled upon the answer to the buildup of greenhouse gases in the atmosphere — and it's been sitting on supermarket shelves all along: baking soda.

The experts developed a new type of carbon capture medium consisting of core-shell microcapsules that are made up of a highly permeable polymer shell. That shell contains a solution of sodium carbonate, the main ingredient of baking soda — and it can absorb carbon dioxide. The microcapsules have been used in the past for controlling the delivery and release of a

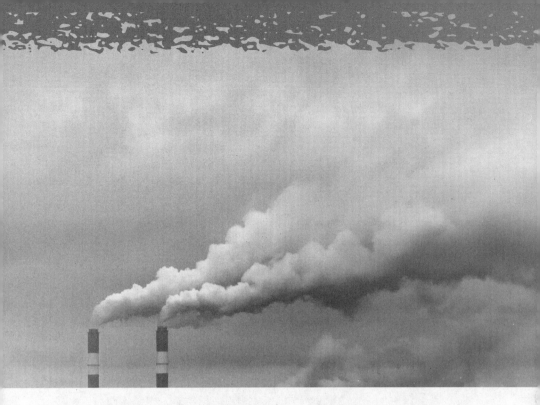

variety of substances, including pharmaceuticals, cosmetics and food flavorings, but this was the first time it was applied to carbon capture. Previous methods were believed to have a negative impact on the environment because of the use of caustic fluids. However, this approach using simple baking soda is not only effective without that, it may simultaneously reduce CO_2 in our planet's atmosphere.

The researchers, whose results were published in the journal _Nature Communications_, say they hope this "breakthrough technique" will eventually be designed to work with power plants run by coal or natural gas as well as other industrial processes, like the production of steel.

Whether or not scientists have found the solution to the carbon emission problem, and we're hoping they have, there's no doubt that using baking soda in your own home can have a positive impact on the environment right now.

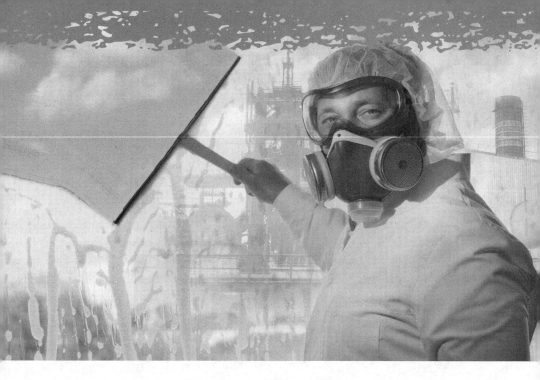

How Baking Soda Can Help Protect the Environment

Baking soda can be used to replace many potentially hazardous household cleaning products that are known to contribute to environmental damage. The majority of store-bought cleaners are loaded with dangerous chemicals. In fact, the average household contains some 62 toxic chemicals, according to <u>environmental experts</u>. We're exposed to them regularly, and so is our environment.

The <u>chemicals in many cleaners</u> are common pollutants that contribute to smog, hurt the quality of drinking water and are toxic to animals too. When they're released into the air, they contribute to pollution. When they're poured down the drain, they seep into the water system. This produces toxic reproductive effects on aquatic species in addition to adversely affecting the water we drink, contributing to climate change and damaging precious ecosystems.

Replacing Standard Household Cleaners With Baking Soda

By using baking soda instead of those chemical-filled household cleaners, you can have a positive impact on saving our environment, and you and your family's health at the same time. These are just a few of the practically endless options for utilizing baking soda to clean your home.

A deodorizer. Arguably the most common use for baking soda in the home is as a deodorizer. It serves to neutralize and buffer, working incredibly well on acidic odors — like those found in your refrigerator. It can also be used in many other places throughout the home. Instead of chemical-filled carpet freshener, use baking soda combined with a few drops of your favorite essential oil.

An all-purpose cleaner. Baking soda combined with white vinegar makes for the ultimate all-purpose cleaner. White vinegar helps to keep your home free of mold and excess bacteria, while making sure your place looks sparkling clean. In fact, experts say that using vinegar it is just as effective as chemicals, if not more so. And by combining it with baking soda, it can be used to clean just about anything.

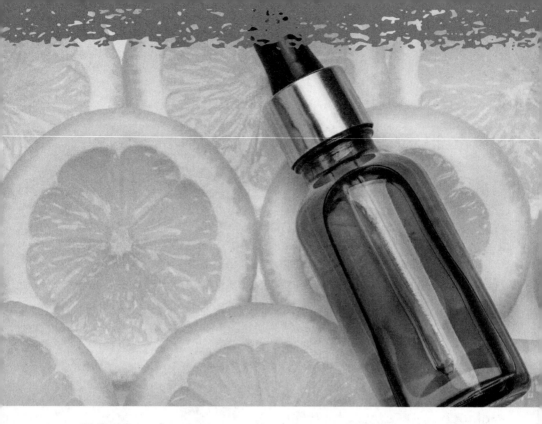

By adding tea tree or lemon essential oil, your homemade cleaner will be able to disinfect, too. To make it, all you need is a spray bottle, a half-cup of white vinegar, two tablespoons of baking soda and ten drops lemon or tea tree essential oil. Add the vinegar and essential oil to the bottle first, followed by the baking soda. Next, add water to fill the bottle to the top and gently shake to mix. When ready to use, simply spray the area you'd likely to clean and then wipe it with a cloth.

Make your silver sparkle again. There's no reason to buy an expensive product that's probably filled with toxins to get your silver sparkling again. Instead, buy non-toxic baking soda for less than a few dollars. To get sterling silver or silverplate pieces nice and shiny, use a baking soda paste made from three parts baking soda to one part water. Rub onto your silver using a clean cloth or sponge, then rinse thoroughly and dry.

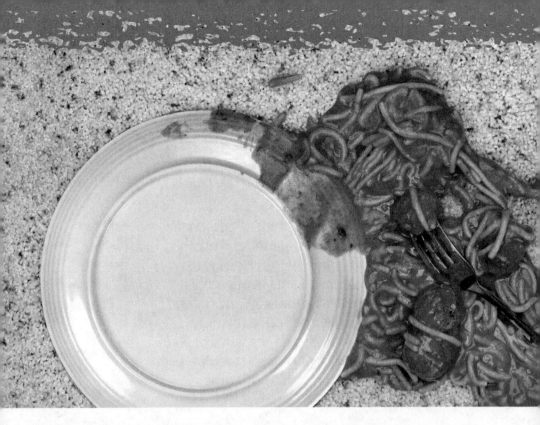

Carpet stain remover. You can even remove stubborn carpet stains with a homemade cleaner that includes baking soda. All you need is enough baking soda to cover the stain, a tablespoon of liquid dishwashing soap, a tablespoon of white vinegar and two cups warm water. Sprinkle the stain with baking soda and then let it sit for ten minutes or so. In the meantime, combine the dish soap, white vinegar and water together in a bowl. Vacuum the baking soda up and then sponge the soap/vinegar/water mixture onto the stain; blot using a dry cloth. Repeat until the stain disappears.

Replacing Personal Care Products with Baking Soda

Most of us have quite an assortment of personal care products in our bathroom cabinets. And according to the Environmental Working Group, one in seven of 82,000 ingredients in personal care products are industrial chemicals, including carcinogens, pesticides, reproductive toxins and hormone disruptors. Not only can these harm your health, but they hurt the environment, too. Instead, replace them by using baking soda with other toxin-free ingredients.

Toothpaste. Using baking soda as part of a homemade toothpaste helps to neutralize acid, whiten teeth, and remove plaque and stains, while coconut oil and tea tree oil offer powerful antibacterial properties. All you have to do is combine the three, using about two tablespoons each of coconut oil and baking soda, and five drops of tea tree oil. You can make a larger or smaller batch depending on the container size you use.

Shampoo. Baking soda even works wonders as a shampoo. It will help remove buildup from styling products and give you more manageable hair. Simply wet your hair and sprinkle a tablespoon onto your scalp. Massage it into your roots and rinse just like you would with traditional shampoo. Following that with an apple cider vinegar rinse will help balance the alkalinity of baking soda, aid in buildup removal and close the hair cuticles. Pour about half a cup of apple cider vinegar over your hair after the baking soda shampoo treatment, then rinse.

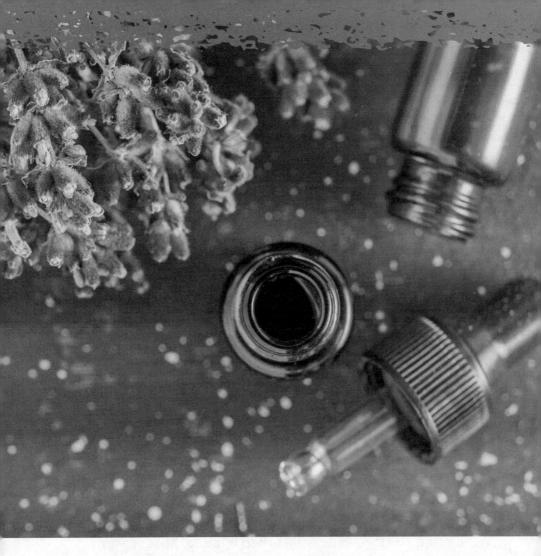

Deodorant. As baking soda is alkaline, it helps to balance out the acids in sweat that encourage bacteria to thrive. It reduces the pH level in areas of the body that commonly sweat, and it counteracts acids to serve as a natural deodorant by absorbing odors. To use it, simply combine half a cup of cornstarch, half a cup of baking soda, and two or three drops of lavender essential oil. Clean your underarms thoroughly, then apply the mixture using a slightly damp cloth and allow it to dry.

Pets and Baking Soda

Just like our personal care products, most conventional store-bought products for pets are filled with potentially harmful chemicals. And, just like us, a dog's skin is its largest organ. In fact, anything you use on their skin and coat can be absorbed into the bloodstream.

Rather disturbing is the fact that when the Environmental Working Group tested 20 dogs and 40 cats in 2008 for chemical contaminants, the animals tested positive for 48 out of 70 industrial chemicals. What makes it even worse is that our furry best friends are even more sensitive to environmental contaminants than we are. This research revealed that average levels of chemical contaminants were much higher in dogs and cats than in humans. The dogs tested 2.4 times higher for perfluorochemicals, while the felines tested five times higher for mercury and 23 times higher in fire retardants.

Cleaning Products, Shampoos, Flea Repellents and Beyond

Certain types of chemical cleaning products, including those we use to clean up our dogs' messes, can put them at risk for organ damage as well as developing allergies, anemia and even cancer. Even after the use of chemical cleaners, residual vapors can linger behind, posing a threat to both animals and humans.

The EWG reports that the researchers in the 2008 study found that the urine and blood samples of dogs contained 11 carcinogens, 31 chemicals toxic to the reproductive system and 24 neurotoxins. The carcinogens, they note, are of particular concern as dogs have much higher rates of many kinds of cancer than people do, including 35 times more skin cancer, four times more breast tumors, eight times more bone cancer and twice the incidence of leukemia. Cancer is one of the most common causes of death in dogs.

Even dog shampoos are risky; take a look at the ingredient list on the label. Odds are, there are lots of hard-to-pronounce names. Plus, those labels are often filled with tricky definitions that make it difficult to determine what to look for. The same ingredient can be classified as a mild skin irritant or one that's known to cause cancer, depending on the manufacturer's process. Making things even more complicated is that many of those manufacturers purchase the source ingredients and then combine them to develop their product. Of course, the manufacturer of your four-legged friend's shampoo probably isn't buying coconut oil and synthesizing it to develop sodium lauryl sulfate. They're likely purchasing sodium lauryl sulfate and mixing it with other chemicals in order to develop their final formula.

And, what about flea repellants? Would you really spray pesticide directly onto your fur baby? Of course not. Yet, many of us do just that, directly applying flea repellents, collars and other chemical products marketed to protect them against ticks and fleas.

Countless Unnecessary Deaths Related to Insect Repellant Products

The Natural Resources Defense Council reports that hundreds (and possibly thousands) of dogs have become ill or died from pesticide exposure related to flea and tick products. In 1988, Hartz flea products were said to be the cause of at least 200 deaths, and thousands more in 2002. More recently, a flea killer called Bravecto was blamed for 355 deaths since its release in 2014, and European regulators have linked it to over 800 pet deaths worldwide.

How Baking Soda Can Help

Isn't it about time that you considered much safer alternatives for all of the products you use on your dog, as well as the product's he's exposed to? Baking soda is ideal — this miraculous substance can be utilized for a myriad of different things, and a box of the stuff is probably in your kitchen cabinets right now. Unlike those products that contain a host of potentially toxic chemicals or fragrances, it contains no harmful chemicals and poses no danger to animals or humans, unless ingested in very large amounts.

Ways to Use Baking Soda as a Healthier, Effective Alternative

Killing Fleas

No matter what those advertisers say, there is no magic formula for controlling fleas on Fido. They may insist their formulas are safe and 100 percent organic, but there is no chemical compound that actually exists which can control fleas and leave your household completely safe. Baking soda, however, can be used along with table salt as a safe, inexpensive option for successfully controlling fleas. It works by getting rid of their larvae and eggs.

When using baking soda to kill fleas, make sure that the product you have is still active. Many of us probably have one or more very old boxes sitting on our shelves. To test the baking soda, simply add a few drops of vinegar to it. The mixture should bubble as soon as it's added, and continue to do so for several minutes. If bubbles don't form, or form very slowly, you need some new baking soda for it to be effective.

In order to kill those fleas, you'll need to treat bedding, carpets and furniture, otherwise the fleas will just continue to thrive and multiply on their favorite breeding grounds. That means you'll need a lot of baking soda, so just one little box isn't going to cut it. Think *gallons* of the stuff, along with gallons of salt. This is particularly true when you have a large home, in which treating all of the rooms is important for eradicating an infestation.

Here's how to do it:

1. Keep your furry friends outdoors or in another safe place when you treat your home, as the baking soda/salt can irritate their skin, especially if they have any sores or open wounds.

2. Combine the baking soda and salt, then pour it into a shaker bottle. Or, you can keep the baking soda and salt separate, apply both to furniture, carpets, etc.

3. Liberally sprinkle the baking soda and salt on all areas of the home as mentioned, including carpets, furniture, bedding and so on. Use a brush or broom to make sure that the mixture is spread evenly.

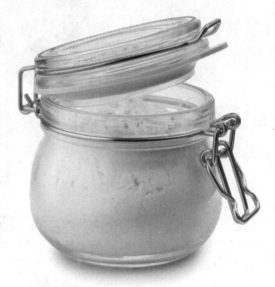

4. Allow the salt/baking soda to remain overnight. It will work to dehydrate fleas and eventually kill them.

5. The following day, vacuum everything up to get rid of dying and dead fleas. If you have a bagged vacuum, be sure to seal the disposable bags and get them outside into a garbage can as quickly as possible.

6. Repeat this process every three to four days, as flea eggs hatch within this period. This will ensure that you eliminate all remaining fleas.

7. Even if there are no signs of fleas in your home anymore, it's best to repeat this process every three months or so to ensure they don't return.

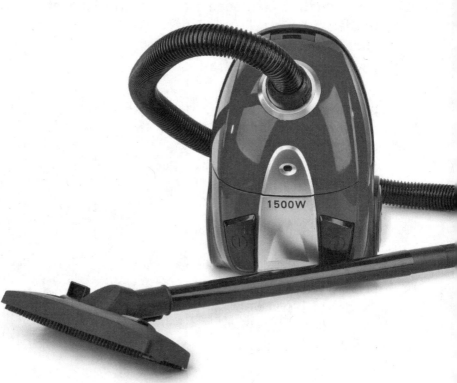

Eliminating Odors

When you have a dog, those dog odors can get pretty nasty, but you can use baking soda to eliminate them. Even if it's a puppy in the process of house training that's making mistakes, sodium bicarbonate is highly effective. That's because the animals' urine is usually acidic, which has a key role in creating a foul-smelling odor. Baking soda is a base, while that urine is acidic. So if you put them together, the baking soda can neutralize that acidic substance, making it more alkaline to eliminate the odor.

No matter what that pet odor is, you can use baking soda to sprinkle on furniture, bedding and carpets to get rid of it. Simply leave it on for 20 to 30 minutes and then vacuum it up. You may want to test a spot first to make sure the baking soda won't discolor upholstery or carpets.

Clean Up an Accident

Of course, the smell isn't the only concern when Fluffy or Fido make a mistake, something that's not only common in puppies, but in dogs that are ill or elderly, and you'll want to get it cleaned up as quickly as possible to prevent a stain. To do so, first apply a little club soda to the mess, leaving it until it's thoroughly dry. Afterwards, sprinkle baking soda on the area and allow that to sit for about half an hour before vacuuming it up.

Clean and Deodorize Bedding

Your dog's bedding can get especially dirty and smelly for obvious reasons — he probably spends a lot of time there. Instead of using harsh chemical detergents, use a mild laundry detergent combined with a cup of baking soda in your washing machine to wash the bedding. If your furry friend spends time in your bed, when you wash your sheets, add half a cup of baking soda to the washing machine to neutralize any odor.

Remove that Awful Skunk Smell

If your dog has an encounter with a skunk, that's a whole new level of foul. The odor can be downright nauseating and difficult to get rid of. Unfortunately, living in many rural areas, that's simply a part of life. The good news is that you don't need to resort to chemicals to get rid of this either. Baking soda can help, along with hydrogen peroxide and some mild dishwashing detergent.

Ingredients

- 1 quart hydrogen peroxide
- 1/4 cup baking soda
- 1 tsp mild dishwashing detergent

Combine the hydrogen peroxide, baking soda and dishwashing detergent in a container like a bucket and then put your dog in the bathtub. Or, to avoid the odor from permeating throughout your house, bathe him outside using a hose. If your dog was sprayed in the face, you can use it to wash this area, but use a small towel to gently apply it, avoiding his eyes, nose and mouth.

Use the mixture just like you would a dog shampoo, lathering up and rinsing well afterwards. If any bedding or clothing soaked up the smell, you can use this same solution to wash it. You may have to bathe your dog with it a couple more times to completely get rid of the odor, but even after the first wash, you'll notice significant improvement. Ideally, repeat the process once the same day, and then once a week for the next couple of weeks.

Give Fido a Dry Bath

If you don't have time to bathe your cuddly best friend and he's just come in from outside after rolling in something yucky, you can use baking soda to give him a dry bath. First, be sure that his fur is totally dry, and then sprinkle the white powder lightly over his coat. Gently rub it in and brush it through. It will relieve itching and help make him more presentable until you can actually get him into that tub for a bath.

Clean Dog Toys

Those dog toys get pretty gross, with your canine putting them through all sorts of torture that can result in dirt, drool and what-have-you all over them. Instead of using a chemical household cleaner, dissolve four tablespoons of baking soda into one quart of water. Using an old toothbrush, dip it into the mixture and use it to scrub the toys. For stuffed toys that aren't meant to get wet, sprinkle the surface with baking soda, leave it for 15 to 20 minutes, then brush it off.

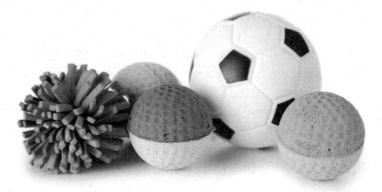

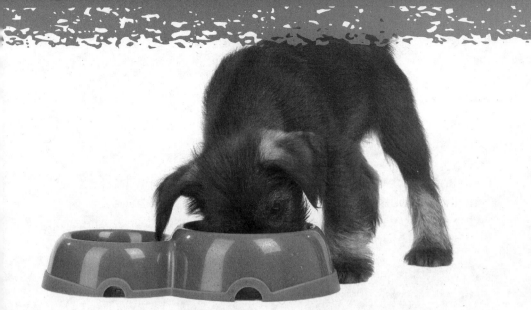

Clean Food and Water Bowls

To keep your pet's plastic, ceramic or stainless steel food and water bowls clean, you can use baking soda, combined with salt and some water. This simple solution helps to scrub off that hard-to-get food and grime. Plus you can use it to clean many other surfaces, like countertops, cutting boards and so on.

To make it, combine equal parts of baking soda, warm water and salt, creating a thick paste. Apply some of the paste using a sponge or cloth to scrub the inside and outside of the piece you want to clean, using a circular motion. Rinse well using warm water.

Relieve the Pain of a Bee Sting

Baking soda is ideal for treating painful bee stings, whether it's an animal or a human who is unlucky enough to get stung. Simply create a paste using baking soda and water to place on the affected area. If the stinger is still inside the skin, use tweezers to try and remove it before applying the paste, if you can.

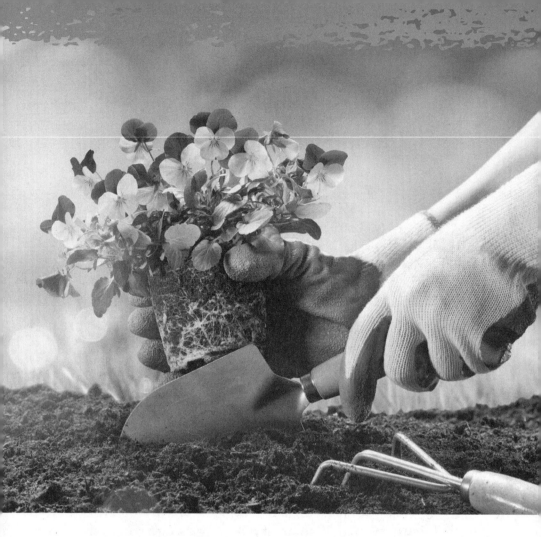

Gardening and Baking Soda

Every year there are 136 million pounds of <u>pesticides</u> used on North American gardens and lawns. Surprisingly, homeowners are reported to use about three times the amount of pesticides as farmers. In fact, the majority of wildlife poisoning and water contamination is not from farms or other large organizations — it's from single-family homes!

Traditional gardening products, including chemical treatments like insecticides and pesticides, come with some serious risks, to humans, pets, wildlife and the environment. According to Environment and Human Health, Inc. (EHHI), the Environmental Protection Agency has approved over 200 different pesticides for lawn care, but they're frequently combined with and sold with other toxic chemicals. Then there are those common chemical-filled cleaners that many of us use throughout our homes and outdoors. Here are just some of the dangers of all of these chemicals:

Harming drinking water. Chemicals leach into surface and groundwater, which in turn harms the quality of our drinking water as well as the quality of aquatic habitats and health of aquatic life forms.

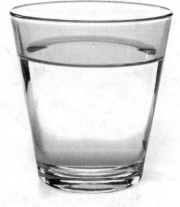

Threatening our children's health. These chemicals are especially hazardous to children's health. They're particularly vulnerable due to their small size and underdeveloped physiology. They're also more often exposed to pesticides due to their behaviors, like playing on grass and putting toys into their mouth.

Threatening the health of our pets. When your pets go outside, they can be exposed to chemicals in the garden and yard. Exposure can also occur because of their behavior as well, such as licking paws that have been contaminated, eating the grass, soil and so on. They're also much more vulnerable to side effects because of their smaller size.

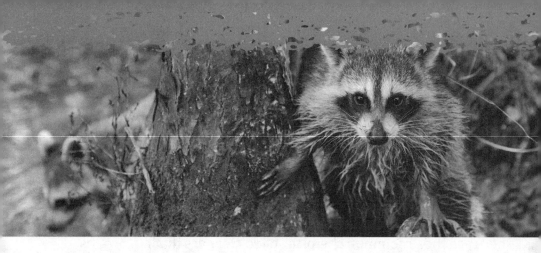

Wildlife is threatened. Local wildlife is at risk too, including animals like raccoons, deer, squirrels, Canada geese and all types of other birds.

Harming beneficial organisms. Chemicals can also threaten the lives of beneficial organisms such as earthworms which kill pests, halt the spread of disease and aid plants in gathering water and nutrients. These pesticides also decrease activity levels which in turn negatively impacts a lawn's natural ability to control diseases and pests, gather water and nutrients, and maintain overall health.

Degrading the overall health of your garden and yard. Applying pesticides on a regular basis creates a chemical-dependent landscape. When pest species become resistant to the chemicals that are meant to eradicate them (a common occurrence), larger, more concentrated doses and more frequent applications become necessary. That results in a never-ending cycle of greater pest resistance and pesticide use, while seriously harming the health of your lawn and garden.

So, what can you use instead?

You might be surprised to learn that the famous little orange box of baking soda in your fridge can work wonders when it comes to everything from helping plants thrive to cleaning and even pest control, without those harmful side effects.

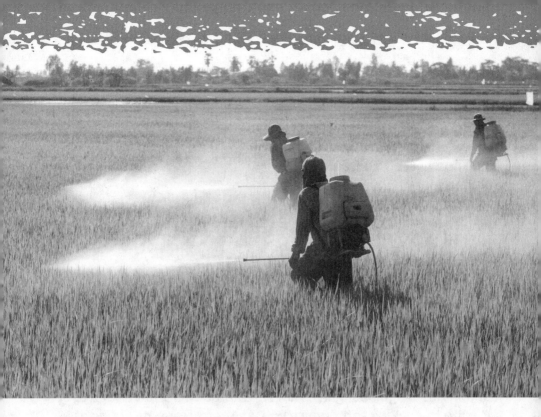

An Alternative Pesticide

Baking soda makes for a totally safe and effective, organic pesticide spray that can eradicate the insects that might harm your plants, like spider mites and aphids, all without negatively impacting us, our planet, wildlife or the plants themselves in the process. Plus, it's a lot less expensive than those chemical sprays!

Combine a teaspoon of baking soda and a third of a cup of olive oil. After you mix it together, add one cup of water. Combine thoroughly and then add the solution to a spray bottle. If your plants are suffering from any type of fungal disease, you can also use it to spray affected areas, spraying every three days until the problem has resolved. It's great on roses that have black spot fungus, as well as grapes and vines that are sprayed when the fruit first begins to appear.

For an insect infestation, combine two
tablespoons of baking soda, a
tablespoon of olive oil, and a three
or four drops of liquid Ivory
soap into one gallon of water.
Add it to a spray bottle and
spray once every few days to
eliminate harmful insects and
to prevent them from returning.

An ant problem can be halted by going to the source — the ant hill.
All you need is baking soda, some confectioners sugar and vinegar.
Just add five heaping teaspoons of confectioners sugar to a bucket or
other container. You don't have to measure everything out precisely,
just don't use regular sugar, as ants are actually clever enough to
separate the baking soda, which will kill them, from the grains of
regular sugar, but they aren't able to do that with powdered sugar.
Add an equal amount of baking soda to the powdered sugar and
then thoroughly combine the two together. It's effective because the
ants are attracted to the sugar, which they'll eat, and in the process,
consume the baking soda, which is fatal. Add about a teaspoon of
water to the mixture, just enough to make it damp, and then pour it
all over the ant hill.

After you pour the mixture over the ant hill, add a little bit of white
vinegar or apple cider vinegar. That is guaranteed to wipe out any
ants that aren't eradicated by the baking soda, as either type of
vinegar contains insecticidal and fungicidal properties that are
deadly to the tiny creatures.

Revive Lifeless Plants

If your plants are looking tired and lifeless, you can help revive them by watering them with a mixture of one gallon of pure, filtered water, a teaspoon of baking soda, a teaspoon of Epsom salt and half a teaspoon of ammonia. Give each plant about one quart each. The solution acts as a fertilizer to perk up plants and help encourage growth. It's particularly good for rose bushes — you'll be surprised at just how quickly they become more lustrous and vibrant! Aim to use this method once a month to keep your plants thriving.

Get Rid of Weeds and Crabgrass

Weeds have deep roots and can be really difficult to remove or kill completely. But by simply heading to your pantry you can avoid pesticides and use that box of baking soda to inexpensively, and more easily, eradicate them. Whether the weeds or crabgrass are growing in your garden beds, in cracks on sidewalks or patios, baking soda is highly effective. It can kill small weeds that have already sprouted, as well as prevent new weeds from coming up. It burns that unwanted foliage, resulting in weeds disappearing within only a few days. Simply pour a thick layer of baking soda onto the weeds or crabgrass after moistening them with water. Sweep the baking soda into a thick layer and get it inside any concrete cracks.

One thing to keep in mind when using baking soda for this purpose, or any other, is to avoid getting it onto grass and plants that you want to keep. Too much baking soda can burn and even kill them.

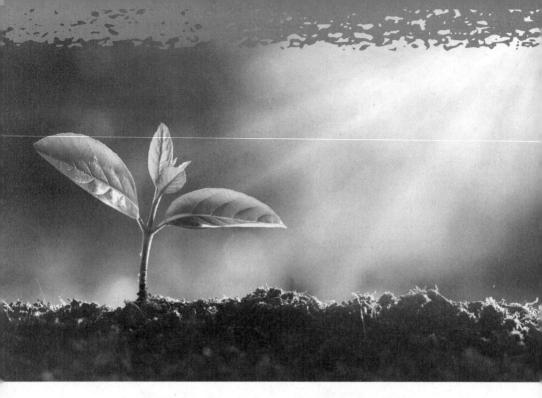

Test the pH of Your Garden Soil

Your garden plants absorb minerals from the soil through their roots, and if that soil is too alkaline or too acidic, that process can be hampered, which is why knowing your soil's pH is so important. You'll be able to find out whether essential minerals will be available to get to the roots of your plants, which is something that's a must for their survival.

The San Francisco Chronicle reports that if you live in an area with alkaline soil, which means it has a pH that's above 7.0, you have two options. Those options are to "either take measures to lower the pH, or you can choose plants well-suited to growing in alkaline conditions. If you take the latter path, you have a wide variety of plants to choose from."

To get an idea of your soil's pH, you can use a mix of baking soda and white vinegar. Start by collecting a couple of soil samples in small cups from different areas of your garden. You'll need a half-cup of baking soda and a half-cup of white vinegar as well.

First, pour the vinegar into one of the soil samples. If the soil starts to bubble, that means it's alkaline, or has a pH level that's higher than 7. If you don't see a reaction, use your other sample and pour in the baking soda and about a half-cup of water. If the soil bubbles, the pH level is below 7, and it is acidic soil.

While you won't get an exact pH level number, this technique is quite helpful when you're faced with trying to make the best decisions about which plants will thrive in your soil, or if you'd like to amend the soil in order to make it more hospitable for your particular gardening goals.

Treat Tomato Diseases

Making a spray using baking soda and aspirin can help treat tomato diseases, including fungal infections and other problems common in tomato plants. Combine two tablespoons of baking soda into two gallons of water in a large spray bottle and then add two aspirin. Mix it together and allow it to sit for several minutes so that the aspirin dissolves. Shake to combine, then spray on affected areas.

Grow Sweeter Tomatoes

In addition to treating tomato diseases, you can make those tomatoes sweeter simply by lowering the acidity of the soil with baking soda. This will also help to discourage any pests. Lightly sprinkle some baking soda onto the soil the tomato plants are in, and it will be absorbed into it, reducing the acidity level of the soil, resulting in tomatoes that have more of a sweet (rather than tart) flavor.

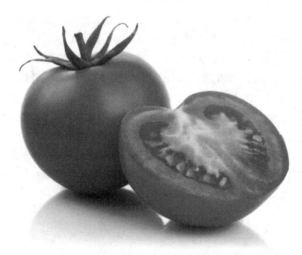

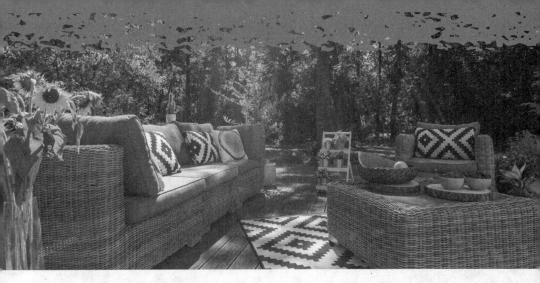

Deodorize Your Compost Bin or Pile

Compost can get awfully smelly, but you can help eliminate that odor by adding a tablespoon of baking soda to a gallon of water. Pour the mixture over the compost to deodorize it. Alternatively, you can sprinkle the dry powder over your compost. With either method, be careful not to overdo it as too much baking soda can slow down composting.

Clean Garden and Patio Furniture

There's no need to use chemical sprays or other solutions for cleaning your outdoor furniture. You can make it look nearly as good as new using baking soda. Simply combine a half-cup of baking soda and a tablespoon of dish soap in a gallon of very warm, almost hot, water. Use the scrubbing side of a sponge to dip into the mixture and then scrub the items you want to clean. Afterward, rinse them using your garden hose.

If you have furniture that's made of webbing material, rinse it off first using your hose, then sprinkle baking soda across it. Let the baking soda sit for several minutes before scrubbing it off and rinsing again.

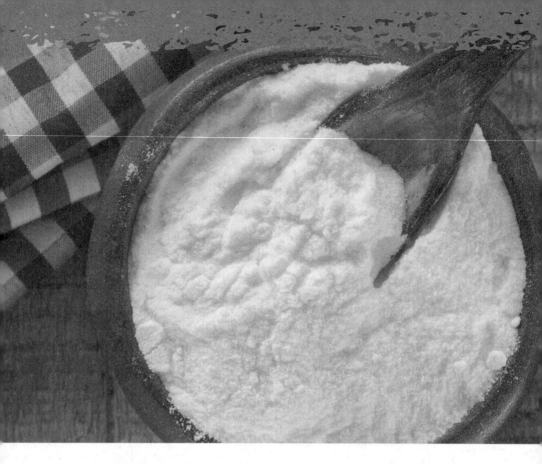

Cooking with Baking Soda: Tips and Tricks

Baking soda isn't just great for deodorizing, it offers many uses in cooking as well. It's a leavening agent most often used in baking to make food rise by releasing carbon dioxide bubbles that expand the dough and create a fluffy result. It forms the texture for cakes, breads, pancakes and many other foods.

In addition to being a common ingredient in lots of baking recipes, baking soda has multiple other culinary uses as well. Here are some tips and tricks for cooking with baking soda that might just be a game-changer in your kitchen.

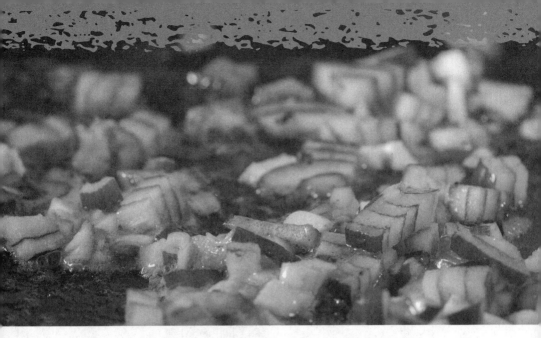

Brown Onions Faster

It can take hours to get beautifully caramelized onions, but you can brown them faster by using baking soda. All you need is a quarter teaspoon for every one pound of sliced onions. In just minutes, they'll be browned as if you'd caramelized them for hours. This isn't a good technique for onions you are planning to use as a burger topping or in a batch of French onion soup, but it's ideal when you want to brown them quickly and use them in a recipe with other ingredients, such as a French onion dip, significantly cutting down your cooking time.

Get Crispier Chicken

You can rub the skin of a chicken with baking soda before you cook it in order to keep the skin nice and crispy while locking moisture in. Simply dust the chicken with a little bit of baking soda and rub it in before seasoning. Then, just slide it into the oven and bake as usual.

Counteract a Too-Strong Vinegar Taste

It's easy to accidentally add a little too much vinegar when following a recipe. Fortunately, baking soda can come to the rescue by counteracting the vinegar taste. Just add a bit of baking soda and the taste won't be as overpowering. Be sure to make that a very tiny amount, as adding too much baking soda to a recipe with vinegar means it will react and start to foam.

Bake Beans That Minimize Gas Production

If you like beans but aren't fond of their effects on your digestive system, just add a little baking soda to the beans as they cook. Their gas-producing properties will be dramatically reduced.

Make Softer Beans to Use in Hummus

Soft beans don't sound all that desirable. In fact, you might think "yuck." But soft beans are essential for homemade hummus that's smoother than any store-bought version. The key to getting them that way is to use baking soda. Adding baking soda to the cooking liquid helps to raise its pH, helping beans like chickpeas break down and tenderize more easily.

For cooking a cup of dried beans, dissolve a teaspoon of baking soda in six cups of cold water. Leave it overnight and then refresh both the water and baking soda afterwards. It won't be long before you're enjoying a super silky, especially flavorful bowl of hummus.

Make Fluffier Omelets

You can make your omelets fluffier by adding a half-teaspoon of baking soda for every three eggs that you use.

Lighter, Softer Waffles

Add just an inch of baking soda to any buttermilk waffle recipe in order to create lighter and softer waffles.

Tenderize Meat and Poultry

Chinese cuisine often includes baking soda as a key ingredient to ensure tender meat and poultry. Take a tip from the Chinese and sprinkle some baking soda on small pieces of meat like beef and pork, then place it in your refrigerator for one to two hours to tenderize it. Afterwards, rinse the baking soda off and cook as usual.

For poultry, you can tenderize it by rubbing the cavity with a little baking soda and then putting it in the fridge overnight.

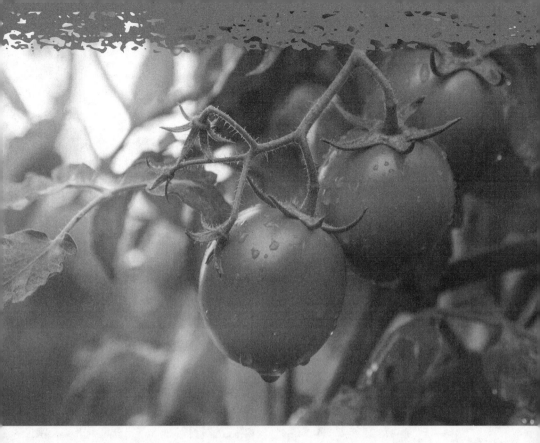

Reduce the Acidity of Tomatoes

Canned tomatoes are something just about all of us have in our pantry, as they can be used in a myriad of different recipes. Unfortunately, the acidity of canned tomatoes can vary significantly depending on the brand, making it hard to know what you're going to have to deal with. The good news is that a quarter teaspoon of baking soda can help, as it functions to neutralize excess acidity, but it won't impact the overall flavor or texture of the tomatoes. In fact, it's said to be the key to smoothing out the flavors in a rich, hearty tomato soup, and pretty much any puree, sauce or chili that's made from an extra-acidic batch of canned tomatoes.

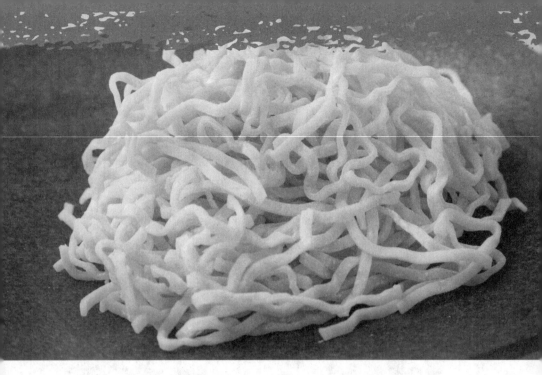

Transform Angel Hair Pasta
Into Ramen Noodles

Have you ever been stuck at home, sick and craving ramen noodles? That's usually the time that it happens, and not the best time to make a trip to the store. While it may sound a bit crazy, baking soda really can help you transform that angel hair pasta into ramen noodles, almost like magic.

Substituting ramen noodles for pasta just isn't the same. But if that happens again, you'll know what to turn to: that little orange box with the white powder. It works because ramen noodles have a springier, stronger texture than spaghetti pasta, and a distinct savory taste due to alkaline elements like kansui, which is usually added to ramen dough. Of course, that's not exactly something that's easy to find. But in this case, baking soda, which is alkaline, is an excellent alternative. While it's not going to be identical, it will definitely do when you're craving a bowl of ramen.

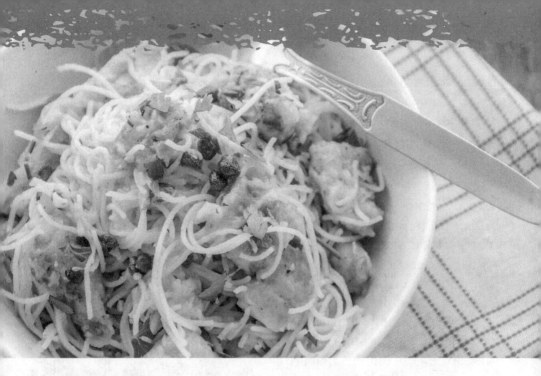

Keep in mind that when you add the baking soda it will cause little foamy bubbles to form, so don't fill your pot all the way to the top. Boil water as though you were making a batch of pasta, in a large pot around two-thirds of the way full. When the water is boiling, add a tablespoon of baking soda.

Don't guess! While adding it in directly from the box, you can easily make the mistake of dumping it in all at once, which will result in a volcano spilling all over your stove. Use a measuring spoon and add it slowly to keep the reaction under control. When the water and baking soda mixture has stopped reacting/foaming, add your pasta, keeping a very close eye on it to prevent an eruption.

Once the pasta is tender, strain it and you'll notice that it's more springy like ramen, and also has more of a yellow hue like ramen, too.

Clarify Iced Tea

Okay, so we know iced tea isn't exactly cooking, but we digress. This is an important summer party trick that can easily earn you the "best host" honor. You can add a pinch of baking soda to brewed tea before chilling it in order to prevent it from turning cloudy. The baking soda will also soften the tannins that are naturally present in tea, giving it a smoother flavor.

Clean Up Your Produce

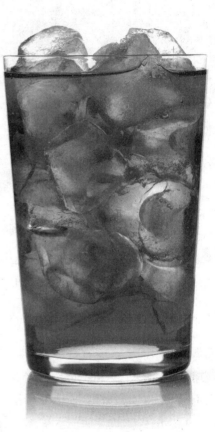

Making sure your produce is thoroughly cleaned is an important part of the cooking process. You can use baking soda to ensure that's accomplished. Just wash your fruits and veggies in a mixture of two to three tablespoons of baking soda and cold water. It will remove impurities left behind by the tap water. You can also use a little baking soda on a wet sponge or a cleaning brush to scrub your produce. Afterwards, be sure to rinse it all thoroughly to get rid of baking soda residue.

Reduce a Fishy Taste

You can even reduce that unpleasant fishy taste by soaking raw fish in a solution of one quart water and two tablespoons baking soda. Let it sit for at least 30 minutes before rinsing it off thoroughly and cooking it.

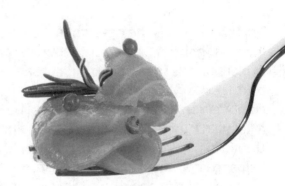

Preparing a Fresh, Whole Chicken

When you need to prepare a fresh, whole chicken, add a teaspoon of baking soda to the water when scalding it so that the feathers will come off more easily. You'll be left with clean, white flesh. Before cooking it, rinse it in cold water and sprinkle baking soda on the inside and the outside, then rinse well.

Soften the Pungent Taste of Wild Game

If you plan to cook wild game, you can soften that pungent taste by soaking it in baking soda and water overnight. Before cooking, rinse it off completely and then dry it.

Improve the Texture of Shrimp

This technique is the best when it comes to improving shrimp, no matter how you plan to cook it. It calls for a quick brine of salt and baking soda. While it may be simple, this combination truly works wonders. The alkaline nature of the baking soda helps to ensure the shrimp have a crisp, firm texture, while the salt helps to keep them nice and moist. You'll need about a teaspoon of salt and a quarter teaspoon of baking soda for every pound of shrimp. Toss it around in the mixture and then place the shrimp in the refrigerator for 30 to 60 minutes.

Neutralize the Acids in a Fruit Recipe

Baking soda can help neutralize the acids in any recipe that calls for a lot of fruit, like cranberry sauce. When you're making it fresh, cover your cranberries with water, and boil them. Then add a tablespoon of baking soda, stir it in, drain the cranberries and then return them to the heat. You'll need less sugar than you usually would to finish the sauce.

For pies and cobblers, you can sweeten tart fruit by adding a half teaspoon of baking soda before adding any sugar. Rhubarb can be soaked in cold water with a pinch of baking soda just before making the sauce.

If you have pineapple that's not quite ripe, you can sprinkle baking soda on it to improve the flavor.

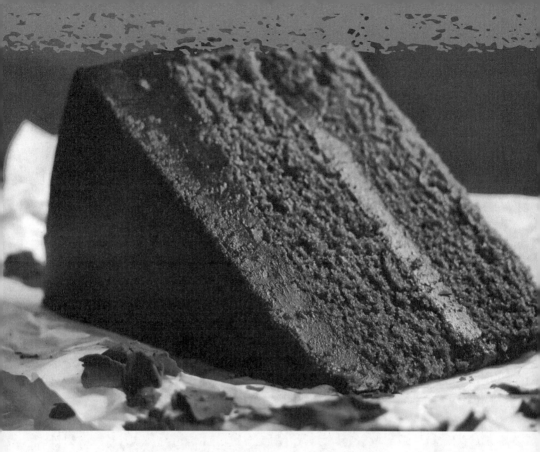

Reduce Acidity in Common Beverages

By adding a pinch of baking soda to a cup of coffee, you can reduce its acidity. If you want to add fizz and reduce acidity in lemonade, grapefruit juice or orange juice, add a quarter teaspoon of baking soda.

Make Chocolate Cake Darker

Add a teaspoon of baking soda to the other dry ingredients in a chocolate cake for a darker colored cake. In a recipe for sour cream cake, combine the baking soda and sour cream before mixing with other ingredients in order to activate the soda more quickly.

Prevent Homemade Frosting From Cracking

Before spreading your homemade frosting on a cake, prevent cracking by adding a pinch of baking soda to it first.

Stop Milk From Curdling When Boiling

When boiling milk on the stove for any recipe, you can avoid curdling by adding a pinch of baking soda. Who knew?

Get Fluffier Rice

When cooking rice, add a teaspoon of baking soda to the water and it will improve its fluffiness.

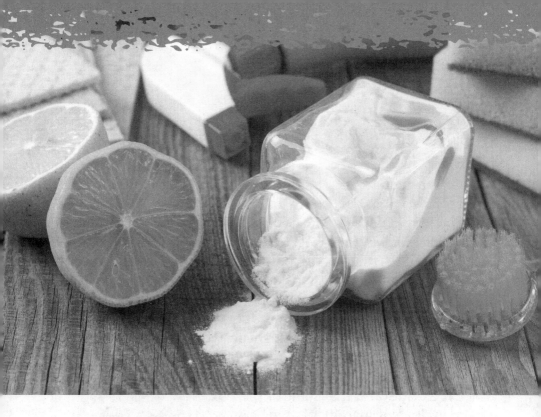

Cleaning With Baking Soda

Many people are making the switch to healthier eating and exercising more regularly, but there is one health topic that is somehow forgotten: chemical cleaning products. While we all want a nice house that's sparkling clean, it's important to be aware that all of those chemicals you're using to make it that way are some of the worst pollutants, harming both human health and the health of the environment.

Just think about the last time you tried to breathe while you were scrubbing the toilet or tub with some chemical spray. If there's no ventilation, it's enough to make you feel as if you're suffocating. And even when there is, a lot of that stuff still gets into your lungs to the point where you're practically gagging.

The Dangers of Chemicals in Traditional Cleaning Supplies

The <u>Environmental Working Group</u> came to a pretty frightening conclusion following an investigation of over 2,000 different cleaning supplies. It notes that "many contain substances linked to serious health problems." One of those issues included asthma induced in otherwise healthy individuals, which was linked to breathing in fumes of some cleaning products, and products containing preservatives that release low levels of formaldehyde, which is known to cause cancer.

The EWG also states that some of the common cleaning ingredients can be laced with the carcinogenic impurity 1,4-dioxane as independent tests have detected the presence of it in multiple name-brand cleaning supplies. In addition, the EWG highlights that studies have found that children born to women who have cleaning jobs while pregnant have a higher risk of birth defects.

Most store-bought household cleaners are filled with harmful chemicals; the average household contains some 62 toxic chemicals, according to a report by <u>environmental experts</u>. That includes everything from noxious fumes in oven cleaners to phthalates in synthetic fragrances.

In a landmark alliance referred to as Project TENDR, leaders of multiple different disciplines came together in a consensus statement noting that many of the chemicals found in everyday products can result in neurodevelopmental disorders, including autism and attention-deficit disorders too.

In 2015, the International Federation of Gynecology and Obstetrics stated: "Widespread exposure to toxic environmental chemicals threatens healthy human reproduction." Other medical groups like the Endocrine Society, the world's oldest and largest organization devoted to researching hormones, have expressed similar concerns.

If you use standard household cleaners, the air in your home may be two to five times more polluted than the air outside. All of those chemicals in the products are the main contributors to indoor air pollution, leading to health problems like asthma as well as dizziness, headaches, fatigue and allergies, not to mention long term health issues that are associated with chronic exposure.

Manufacturers have argued that in small amounts, the toxic ingredients in their cleaners aren't likely to cause problems. But when those products are used on a regular basis, and we're exposed to the chemicals in them regularly, it contributes to the body's "toxic burden," which refers to the amount of chemicals stored in tissues at any given time. That can eventually cause enough harm that it triggers a disease to develop.

Those chemicals also hurt our environment in many different ways as they seep into our water systems and into the air, contributing to air and water pollution. This adversely affects the water we drink, has toxic effects on aquatic species, contributes to climate change and damages precious ecosystems.

Baking Soda: A Better Alternative

Needless to say, the next time your tub is looking a little dirty and you want to scrub it, consider making your own natural cleaning concoction. The same goes for just about anything else in the house, from the refrigerator to the toilet, tub, carpets and even outside on your patio and in your garden. You'd be surprised at what a little baking soda can do — it's not only far cheaper than those chemical cleaners, it's just as effective without the toxic hazards.

If you aren't sure where to start, we'll give you options for every room in the house and then some.

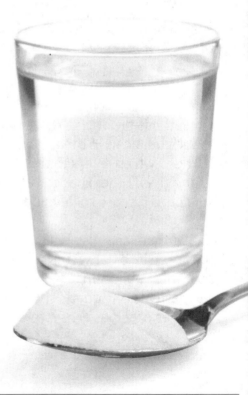

Your Entire Home

All-Purpose Cleaner

It's incredibly convenient to have an all purpose-cleaner that will work on just about every type of surface in your home, and baking soda is an essential non-toxic natural cleaning agent in this recipe that helps to provide scrubbing action and more.

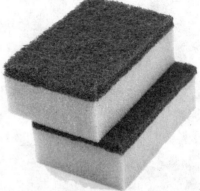

This recipe also calls for white vinegar, one of the most versatile natural cleaning products you can have. It can help keep your home free of mold and excess bacteria, while leaving it sparkling clean. Baking soda and white vinegar make the ideal all-purpose cleaner, and by adding lemon essential oil, it can disinfect too.

Ingredients

- 1/2 cup white vinegar
- 2 tbsp baking soda
- 10 drops lemon or tea tree essential oil

Equipment

- 1 spray bottle

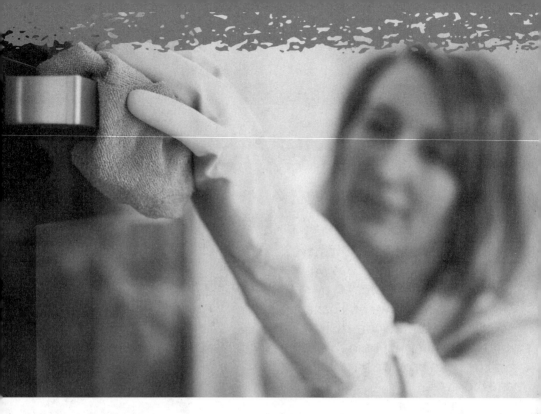

Instructions

1. Add white vinegar and essential oils to your spray bottle.
2. Add baking soda and mix well.
3. Add water to fill the bottle to the top.
4. Gently shake to mix all ingredients.
5. When you're ready to use it, just spray the area you'd like to clean and then wipe it down with a cloth.

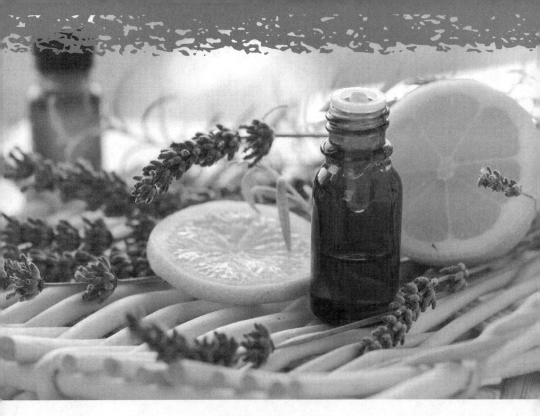

Air Freshener

Baking soda has practically an endless number of uses around the house but it's especially well-known as an odor absorber, which is why it's ideal for a natural alternative to those chemical fresheners.

Ingredients

- Baking soda
- Your favorite essential oils

Equipment

- 1 small glass jar with a vented lid — a half-pint mason jar and a piece of construction paper with a few holes cut out in place of the lid works well

Instructions

1. Fill the jar with baking soda and then add the essential oils, using six drops per tablespoon of baking soda.

2. Place the jar in the room you want to freshen and deodorize the air. You can make several, strategically placing them throughout your home.

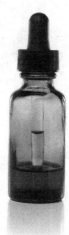

When the baking soda begins to harden, or gets clumpy, it usually indicates that it's absorbed moisture, which means it won't be as effective at neutralizing odors. That's when you'll need to replace it.

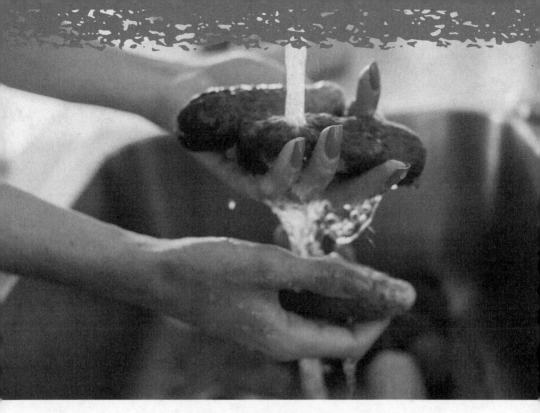

Your Kitchen

When you've got baking soda, there's no need for a cabinet filled with cleaners to deep clean your kitchen or take care of many everyday kitchen tasks either.

Produce Cleaner

Forget about the produce wash. Instead, all you need is a little baking soda and a damp sponge. Use it to scrub your produce, rinse and voila! It's ready to eat.

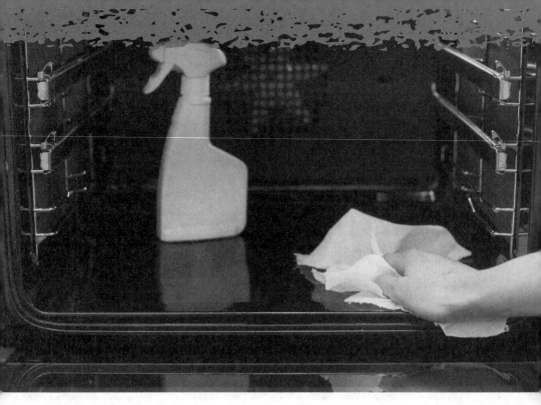

Oven Cleaner

Cleaning your oven can be a challenging task, but it can be accomplished with a little baking soda, elbow grease and a couple of other ingredients.

Ingredients

- Baking soda
- White vinegar
- Water

Equipment

- Protective gloves
- A damp cloth
- Spatula (plastic or silicone)
- Spray bottle

Instructions

1. Empty your oven completely, removing all of the oven racks, pizza stone, thermometer or anything else that you might have in there.

2. Make a baking soda paste by combining a half-cup baking soda with a few tablespoons of water in a small bowl. If the consistency isn't right, adjust the ratio until it becomes more spreadable.

3. Coat your oven with the paste by spreading it all over the interior surfaces, avoiding the heating elements. The gloves are for this step, so you can get into all those nooks and crannies without getting the grime underneath your nails. The baking soda will become a brownish shade as it's rubbed in, and it may be chunkier in some spots, but that's not a problem. Just coat the inside the best you can, paying extra attention to areas that are especially greasy.

4. Allow your oven to sit like this with the baking soda mixture for at least 12 hours, or overnight.

5. Now it's time to work on your oven racks. Sprinkle them with baking soda and then spray them with vinegar. Once the foaming stops, submerge them in a tub of hot water and allow them to sit for at least 12 hours, or overnight.

6. In the morning, scrub the grease and grime off the racks using an old dish towel. If there's really stubborn grime, use an old toothbrush to dislodge it. Afterwards, rinse them off and set them aside.

7. Now get to the interior of your oven, using your damp dish cloth to wipe out as much of the dried baking soda paste as possible, using the spatula to help scrape off the paste as you need to.

8. Put the vinegar into a spray bottle and spray everywhere there is baking soda residue in the oven. It will react with the baking soda and gently foam.

9. Wipe down the oven again, using your damp cloth to get the foamy vinegar-baking soda mixture. Repeat until all of the residue is gone. If you need to, add a bit more vinegar or water while you're wiping it down to help it get nice and shiny.

10. Replace your oven racks and any other items that you keep inside your oven.

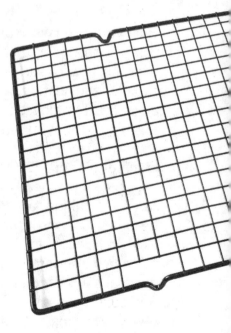

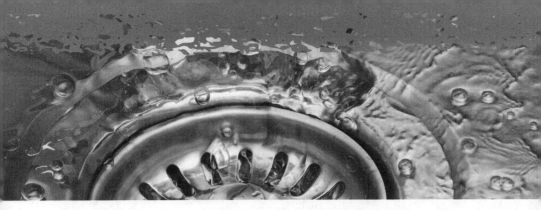

A Drain Cleaner

The main ingredient in most drain cleaners is either sulphuric acid or sodium hydroxide, which can cause serious injury when coming into contact with skin or when ingested, in addition to harming the environment if it is improperly stored or used too often.

Drain cleaners are truly one of the worst — if the chemicals get onto your skin, they can burn. And if some of the solution happens to splash into your eyes, it can even blind you. Plus, the disposal of these solvent-based cleaners can contaminate drinking water and potentially damage septic systems, too.

Instead, use this non-toxic, far less corrosive natural method that utilizes baking soda. Keep in mind that a do-it-yourself solution generally works best when used routinely before a clog occurs. If your drain is already clogged, it will take longer than those toxic commercial cleaners. In fact, you might have to repeat your efforts a few times before it works, but it is well worth the wait.

All you have to do is mix a cup of baking soda with a cup of apple cider vinegar. Pour it down the drain, and you'll see it bubble and fizz. Wait for about a half hour, and then run hot water into the drain. Repeat until the drain is no longer clogged. Aim to do this on a regular basis to prevent clogs from happening in the first place.

Floor Cleaner

Baking soda is also an ideal ingredient in a homemade floor cleaner, helping to scrub those floors until they glisten. This solution, utilizing baking soda, white vinegar, dishwashing detergent and water is strong enough to remove dirt and grime from finished hardwood, vinyl, laminate and porcelain tile.

Combine a half-cup water, half-cup dishwashing detergent, one and two-thirds cups baking soda and two tablespoons of white vinegar. Mix well until all the lumps are dissolved, then pour it into a clean spray bottle. Wash your floor in small sections by spraying on, mopping off, then rinsing thoroughly with clear water. Be sure to rinse, otherwise you'll be left with streak marks on your floor.

If you have darkened, stained grout on your kitchen floor (or other areas like an entryway), it's no match for baking soda and a little scrubbing with a toothbrush. Simply add water to baking soda to achieve a paste and then paint over the grout lines with an old toothbrush. Follow up by applying equal parts of water and vinegar. Allow the mixture to foam and then use the toothbrush to gently scrub. Rinse well afterwards.

If your floor isn't really dirty, just looking dull, you can brighten it up by dissolving a half-cup of baking soda in a tub or bucket of warm water. Mop with this and then rinse with clear water and your floor will be shiny again.

Scour a Ceramic Cooktop

Food residue tends to build up on cooktops and it doesn't seem to matter how often or how hard you work at trying to keep them clean. The good news is that you can mix up a paste, using baking soda and warm water to loosen that gunk up. Allow it to sit for a few minutes after applying, and then scrub it with a clean cloth. Rinse and wipe dry.

Renew Burned Stainless Steel Cookware

All you need to get those blackened, burned stains off stainless steel cookware is baking soda, water and a mesh dish cloth. Place your old pan or pot on a stovetop burner and fill to the top with water. For really tough stains, add a little white vinegar to the water. Bring the water to a boil and allow it to boil for 20 minutes. Afterwards, you'll notice that the staining has become loose; you can test it by lightly scraping with a wooden spoon.

Remove the pot or pan from the heat and pour out the now darkened liquid; that color indicates that the process is working. Coat the bottom of the pot or pan with baking soda and then scrub it with your mesh dish cloth. Rinse well. It will be shiny and almost like new!

Make Your Silver Sparkle Again

Baking soda is the best for polishing silver without harmful chemicals. To shine your sterling silver or silverplate pieces, combine three parts of baking soda to one part water, forming a paste. Rub the paste onto your silver using a clean cloth. Rinse thoroughly afterwards and allow it to dry.

Dishwasher Cleaner

You can clean your dishwasher simply by running an empty cycle with baking soda instead of dishwashing detergent.

Refrigerator Cleaner

It doesn't take long for spills, crumbs and other food and drink residue to dirty up your refrigerator, but you can easily remove them using dish soap and baking soda. Combine the two together to make a paste, then use the scrub side of a sponge to eliminate stubborn spots. Wipe it away using warm water.

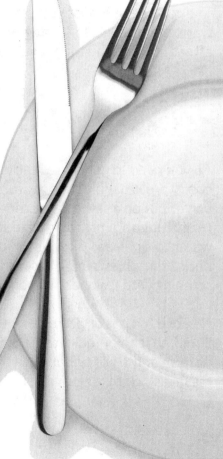

Refreshing Stale-Smelling Sponges

Soak your old sponges in baking soda and water to freshen them up so that they'll last a bit longer. Generally, you should still be tossing them out every few weeks, but if it hasn't been that long, this is a good way to save a little money.

Living Room

Carpet Freshener

To make your carpets or rugs smell fresher, combine a cup of baking soda with two tablespoons of lemon juice. Sprinkle the mixture over your carpets or rugs, allow it to sit for a few minutes, then vacuum it up.

Deodorize Musty Upholstery

After awhile, upholstery can start to develop an unpleasant musty smell. You can banish odors from the soft, cushiony areas by sprinkling them with baking soda, just like your carpet. Allow it to sit for 15 minutes and then vacuum it up.

Remove Grime From Your Couch

If your couch is looking like it belongs out there on a curb with a free sign on it, baking soda might be able to come to the rescue, if it isn't too far gone. All you need is a clean cloth, baking soda and a vacuum with a brush attachment. First, wipe it down using a dry cloth or a stiff brush, to get dried-on gunk and dust off. Sprinkle baking soda on it and allow it to sit for 30 minutes. Now, vacuum the baking soda up using the brush attachment.

Removing Water Stains From Wood Coffee Tables

Baking soda can help remove those stubborn coffee table stains like magic. All you have to do is make a paste with water and baking soda. Dampen a clean cloth with a little water and then add the paste to it. Rub with the grain to buff out the ring and then use a dry cloth to wipe it off.

You may have to repeat a second time, but it will come off.

Bathrooms

Toilet bowl cleaner

Pretty much everything in your bathroom can be cleaned using baking soda too, including that gross toilet bowl. All you need is a cup of baking soda and a cup of white vinegar. First, shut off the flow valve to the toilet and then flush one to two times until the water is drained. Pour in the baking soda and then slowly pour in the vinegar. Make sure that the vinegar covers as much of the bowl surface as possible. If you'd like a fragrance, add ten drops of your favorite essential oil scent. The baking soda will react with the vinegar. Once it does, use a toilet brush to scrub the surface and remove any stains. Turn the water back on and flush.

Shower and Tub Cleaner

Get your tub and shower sparkling clean using a three-quarter cup of baking soda, quarter-cup Castile soap and a tablespoon of water. Place everything into a large bowl and mix it up well. Now, spread the solution onto the areas you'd like to clean, and then rub it in gently using a sponge or rag. Rinse well afterwards.

You can also banish mildew stains by scrubbing your tub, tile, sink and shower curtain with a damp sponge and baking soda. Rinse and a gleaming surface will appear once again.

Glass Shower Doors

While glass shower doors provide an elegant touch to your bathroom, they often end up with water spots, residue from shaving cream and other bath products that are unattractive, detracting from that look you hoped to achieve. Most experts advise against using scouring powders, since those tiny, gritty granules that scrub off strains can also leave tiny scratches.

Fortunately, baking soda is different. It's not only effective, because it's a salt that dissolves in water and the granules are just .0026 inches in diameter, but it also won't harm the glass. All you have to do is sprinkle a little baking soda onto a damp sponge, then wipe down the glass. Rinse with clear water and use a squeegee for an especially sharp finish that won't leave lint and minimizes streaking.

Drains and Faucets

Standing water can mar the shine of chrome — it doesn't leave a stain, rather, it leaves mineral build-up. When there is water pooling around faucets and drains, the minerals tend to settle to the bottom and eventually leave surfaces of the sink or tub with a rough ridge of calcium carbonate, otherwise known as limescale or just lime.

In addition to toxicity concerns, commercial cleansers that are specifically designed to dissolve lime and other mineral deposits come with other negative aspects. They can damage or discolor chrome, stainless steel, brass, bronze and nickel finishes. But once again, it's baking soda— and vinegar — to the rescue.

Vinegar helps to dissolve lime without harming those metal finishes, although it will work more slowly so it needs to be applied continuously. To keep it from running off or drying, that's where baking soda comes in. Mix some with the vinegar, enough to form a paste and then thoroughly coat the lime area. Allow it to sit for several hours and then rinse. If you have heavy deposits of lime, you may need to repeat this two or three times for good results.

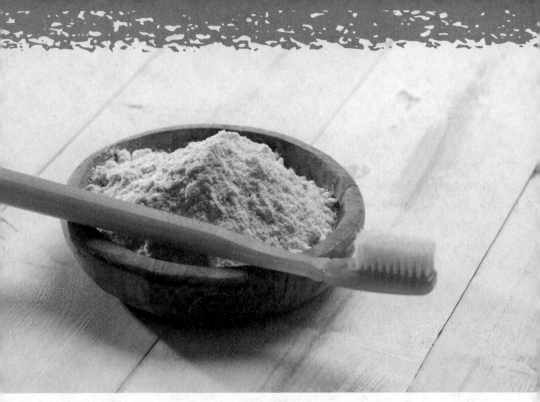

Hair Brush Cleaner

Hair brushes can get dirty quickly with all that product build-up, oils and such. Many people forget about cleaning them, but if you want hair that's shiny and lustrous, your brushes need to be clean. Remove the buildup and residue by soaking your hair brushes in a solution of three tablespoons of baking soda in a small basin of warm water. Rinse and then allow them to dry.

Toothbrush Cleaner

You can clean your toothbrushes by soaking them in a mixture of a quater-cup baking soda and a quarter-cup water. Allow them to soak overnight for a thorough cleaning.

Deodorizing a Front-Load Washer

A front-load washer is more efficient and uses less detergent than traditional top-loading models, but it's more prone to putting off a smelly odor over time. To keep it smelling fresh — and ensure your laundry smells it's best — add a half-cup of baking soda to the detergent cup and then run a wash cycle using hot water. It will deodorize the machine and help cut soap scum, too. Aim to do this deep cleaning once a month to keep it that way.

Keep Linen Closet Odors Away

Just like in the refrigerator and so many other places in your home, you can open up a box of baking soda and leave it near your sheets and towels in the linen closet to help fight musty odors.

Outdoor Areas

Cleaning Dirty Patio Furniture

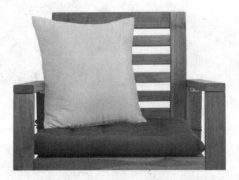

That outdoor patio furniture can get dirty quickly, even when it's stored away. Before you pull it out for the season, give it a good cleanup by wiping all the pieces down with baking soda and water. To help keep them fresh when putting them away again, place baking soda underneath all cushions or inside their storage bags.

Get Rid of Garbage Can Odors

Who wants those garbage smells permeating through the backyard or other areas near the house? It doesn't make dining outside or other activities very pleasant. You can easily get rid of that odor by placing some baking soda in the bottom of each garbage can before tossing in those bags.

Clean Up the BBQ Grill

Here's a great way to get rid of all the grime that comes with cooking on the grill during summer: simply sprinkle baking soda on a grill-cleaning brush before you scrub.

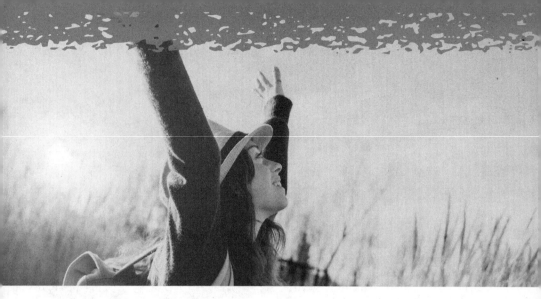

Baking Soda For Your Health

Baking soda is best-known for its cooking purposes. It's used as a leavening agent when making baked goods, and when it's combined with an acid, it reacts, creating bubbles and giving off carbon dioxide gas, which results in the dough rising. It's also commonly used to deodorize the refrigerator, with many a home keeping a box of baking soda opened in the refrigerator.

Numerous anecdotal reports have suggested that multiple forms of 100 percent sodium bicarbonate have been used for centuries, from the Ancient Egyptians who used natural deposits of natron, a mixture containing sodium hydrogen carbonate, as paint for hieroglyphics, treating wounds and to clean their teeth.

In the late 18th-century, sodium carbonate was produced as a leavening agent for home baking, and by the 1860s, it was frequently featured in cookbooks as an additive. By the 1920s, we began to learn about its incredible versatility, and within a decade it was widely advertised as a "proven medical agent."

Today, we know it's good for practically an endless number of things, including enhancing your health.

Get Rid of Ingrown Hairs

You'd probably never think of using baking soda to get rid of those frustrating ingrown hairs. Surprisingly, it's not only effective, it's rather mild, which means it's an especially good choice for those with sensitive skin.

Use baking soda as a paste and it will help keep the follicle from becoming clogged while waiting for the hair to break the surface, and it also aids in easing inflammation. Simply combine just enough baking soda and water to form a paste that can be spread across your skin. Don't make it so thick that it will just fall off, rather just thick enough so that it will adhere to your skin. Before applying it, be sure to wash your hands thoroughly with soap and 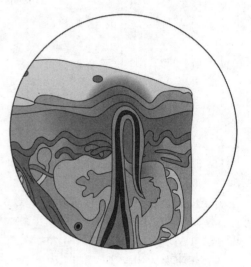 warm water. Apply it by using a firm but gentle circular motion with your fingers. Afterward, rinse with cold water and then apply a small amount of coconut oil to moisturize.

Make a Homemade Deodorant

Most store-bought deodorants contain an ingredient that poses serious risk to one's health: triclosan. It's been shown to alter hormone regulation in addition to contributing to the worldwide problem of antibiotic-resistant bacteria. Other research has found links to weight gain, the inflammatory response, allergies and thyroid dysfunction. Plus, their aluminum compounds are known to block sweat ducts and mimic estrogen which can promote the growth of breast cancer cells.

The good news is that you don't have to give up deodorants completely and live with smelling bad. You can create your own, natural deodorant simply by mixing a teaspoon of baking soda with enough water to create a paste, then rub it on your underarms. For a nice scent, just add a drop or two of your favorite smelling essential oil.

Flu-Proof Frequently Touched Surfaces in Your Room

No one likes to come down with the flu, but given that flu viruses can live for up to eight hours on hard surfaces, lots of people get infected by touching things like germ-filled door knobs and light switches. You can help flu-proof your home by scrubbing surfaces, even hard-to-clean items like your sink using a lemon juice scrub followed with a vinegar spray. Combine a tablespoon of white vinegar with 16 ounces of water in a spray bottle, then dip half of a lemon in baking soda. Use the lemon with baking soda to scrub the item and then spray it using the vinegar spray. Wipe dry with a paper towel.

Sanitize Cutting Boards

Cutting boards are breeding grounds for germs, whether they're made of plastic or wood. The Food Safety Laboratory at the University of California at Davis recommends wood because a knife-scarred plastic cutting board is able to tightly hold onto any bacteria, while a wooden cutting board does not. The downside is that wooden cutting boards can be challenging to clean. Fortunately, the same tough natural cleaning solution as noted above will do the trick. Dip half a lemon in baking soda, then scrub the cutting board directly. Wipe down with vinegar spray and dry with a paper towel.

Control Burping

Some people seem to naturally be chronic burpers, which can be especially embarrassing when you're out in public. If you're a chronic burper, baking soda works as a simple tool for controlling it. Just mix a tablespoon of lemon juice and one-quarter teaspoon of baking soda in a glass of water and drink it after every meal. It will help the digestion process as well as eliminate those burps.

Relieve Acid Reflux and Heartburn Pain

Baking soda contains powerful antacid <u>properties</u>. It is beneficial for relieving indigestion, acid reflux and heartburn along with the common symptoms of peptic ulcer disease. Acidity interferes with the normal digestive process. When an overproduction of stomach acids results from spicy foods, alcohol, overeating, stress and other factors, the acids often go back into the esophagus, which results in acid reflux that causes heartburn.

Frequent episodes can even permanently damage the walls of the esophagus, or worse, trigger cancers. Acidity is often accompanied by other problems like bloating, nausea, indigestion or vomiting. By consuming a baking soda tonic regularly it can help neutralize the effects of acid, supporting better digestion.

Simply mix a teaspoon of baking soda in an eight-ounce glass of water when you're experiencing the pain of heartburn, acid reflux and other digestive ailments.

Halt a Mosquito Bite Itch in its Tracks

Baking soda contains mild alkaline compounds that aid in neutralizing the skin's pH balance, which makes it an outstanding natural remedy for mosquito bites. The baking soda helps to reduce inflammation around the bite which can relieve soreness as well as itching. To use it, mix a tablespoon of baking soda with only enough water to create a paste. Apply the paste to the bite, allowing it to sit for about 10 minutes, then rinse it off.

Relieve Sensitive Teeth

Combined with peppermint oil and coconut oil, baking soda makes an excellent homemade toothpaste that can help relieve sensitive teeth. Peppermint is an antiseptic essential oil that can kill anaerobic bacteria to prevent gum disease as well as help ensure the dentin's protective covering remains intact. Plus, that cool minty flavor makes it the best oil for fighting bad breath. To make it, combine equal parts of baking soda and coconut oil, and then add 10 to 15 drops of peppermint oil.

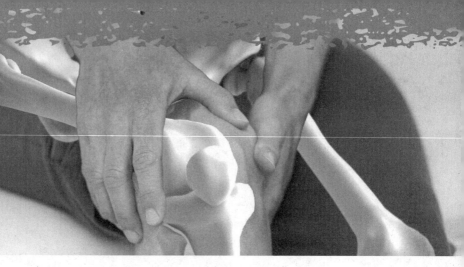

Reduce Inflammation

While apple cider vinegar is popular for easing inflammation and many other benefits, adding baking soda takes its effectiveness up a notch. A tonic of two teaspoons apple cider vinegar and one-eighth teaspoon baking soda combined in an eight-ounce glass of water will help ease joint inflammation and other painful conditions, like gout.

Treat Swollen Feet

When you have to be on your feet for much of the day, they can easily start to swell, something that can be incredibly uncomfortable and even painful. To treat them, fill a foot bath or tub with cool water. You can use any type of container that's at least a foot deep and large enough to hold both feet. Be sure to keep the water more cool than warm, as warm water can increase the swelling and inflammation.

Pour a cup of baking soda into the water and stir to thoroughly combine. Place your feet into the bath and soak them for at least 10 minutes, or however long you need to for relief. If it doesn't seem to be helping, or the water keeps getting warm, you can add ice cubes to the bath.

Prevent Foot Odor and Microbial Infections

Using baking soda combined with essential oils and arrowroot can help protect feet from microbial infections and prevent bad odor, something that's been confirmed in scientific research. The study suggests that making this compound will inhibit yeast, fungal and bacterial growth. Foot odor is caused by warm, moist (as in sweaty) toes and the bacteria that thrive on them. The bacteria grows in this ideal environment created by your feet in shoes.

This foot powder works because baking soda helps to deodorize, and it's also a fungistatic, meaning that bacterial and fungal spores won't be able to germinate (grow) when the alkaline baking soda is present. Sweat is acidic, which is neutralized by alkaline baking soda. Corn starch is highly absorbent, soaking up any moisture left behind, creating a dry environment that's a lot less friendly to fungus and bacteria.

The essential oils in the recipe do more than add fragrance. Tea tree oil has both <u>antifungal</u> and antibacterial properties, as the National Center for Biotechnology Information reports. Eucalyptus provides a fresh, clean aroma as well as containing antifungal and antiseptic properties, while peppermint is soothing and cooling, in addition to offering bacteria-fighting properties.

You can make your own foot powder by mixing the following:

- 6 tsp cornstarch
- 3 tbsp baking soda
- 5 to 10 drops tea tree oil
- 5 to 10 drops eucalyptus oil
- 10 to 15 drops peppermint oil

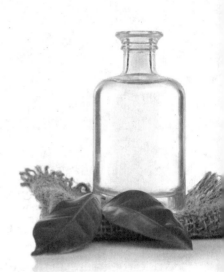

Use the powder by applying it to feet and in between toes. Also sprinkle into your shoes to eliminate odor, leaving it in overnight or longer.

A Foot Exfoliator

You don't have to have swollen feet, an infection or odor to take advantage of baking soda. It can be used as an excellent natural, inexpensive exfoliator. Add three tablespoons of it to a tub of warm water and enjoy an invigorating foot soak. Mix up a thick paste using three parts baking soda to one part water, and scrub your feet with it for added exfoliation. Do this regularly, and you'll have healthy feet that are ready to show off during the warmer months of the year.

Soothe Chafing

A relaxing soak in a tub with the right ingredients, including baking soda, is a fabulous way to soothe irritated, chafed skin too. Just fill a tub with lukewarm water and add two cups baking soda and ten drops lavender essential oil. Soak all affected areas for 15 to 20 minutes, and then gently towel dry. You may want to moisturize using a natural oil, like coconut oil or olive oil, for further relief.

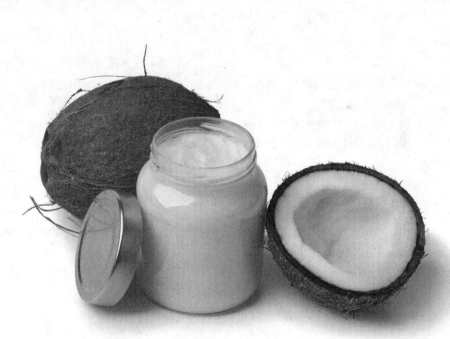

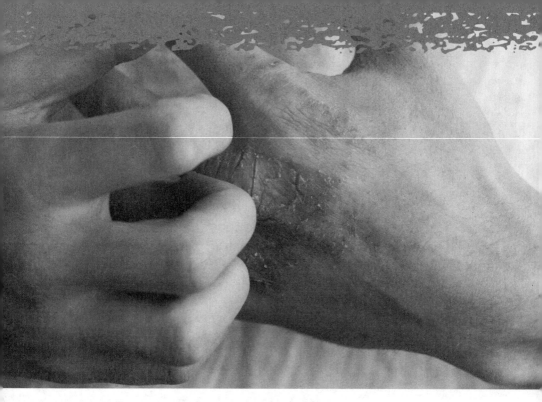

Eczema Relief

Baking soda is great for relieving the pain and itch of eczema too. Assuming that you can physically tolerate being submerged in water during a flare-up, there are several herbs and minerals that you can add to your bath to help clear up and lessen the irritation of eczema rashes. This recipe is ideal for relief and will also help detox your skin:

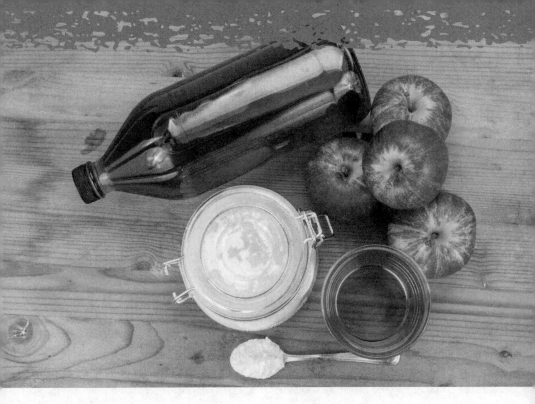

Ingredients

- 1/4 cup Himalayan salt
- 1/4 cup Epsom salt
- 1/4 cup baking soda
- 1/3 cup apple cider vinegar
- 10 drops of your favorite essential oil (lavender, bergamot and chamomile are great)

Instructions

1. Dissolve the dry ingredients, Himalayan salt, Epsom salt and baking soda in boiling water in a quart-size jar and set it aside.

2. Fill a tub with lukewarm water (don't get it too hot or it could irritate skin further) and add apple cider vinegar.

3. Pour salt mixture in, and then add essential oils.

4. Soak for 20 to 30 minutes.

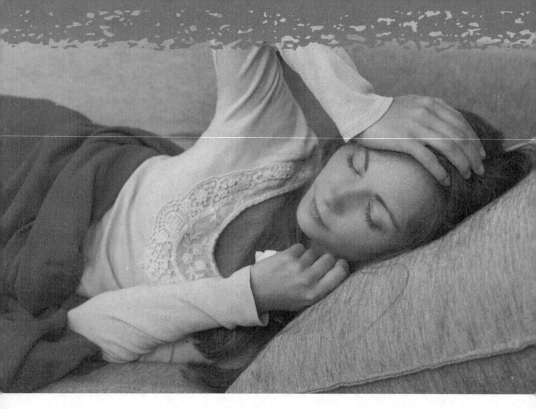

Ease Cold and Flu Symptoms

Baking soda is also great for easing symptoms of a cold, sinusitis or the flu. A saltwater/baking soda wash helps to keep the nasal passages open by washing out thick or dried mucus. It can also help improve the cilia functioning, something that helps keep the sinuses clear. If you have a sinus infection, this helps to prevent the spread of it as well as lessen post-nasal drip while making the nose more comfortable as it keeps mucous membranes moist.

To make it, add a cup of distilled water to a clean container. You can use tap water, but boil it first to sterilize it and then allow it to cool until it's lukewarm. Add a half-teaspoon sea salt to the water followed by a half-teaspoon of baking soda. The solution can be stored at room temperature for three days. Use it two to three times per day, until symptoms have cleared.

Balance pH to Promote Better Health

Keeping your pH balanced is important for promoting better health. If your body is too acidic, it can result in diseases like cancer, arthritis and osteoporosis, as they thrive in an acidic environment. You can use baking soda for this purpose by dissolving one to two teaspoons in a glass of water and drinking the mixture once each day.

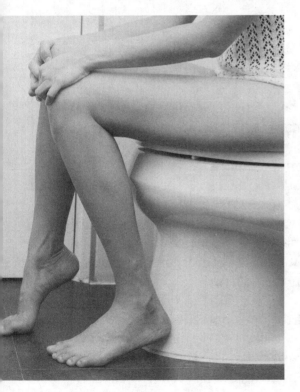

Relieve the Discomfort of a Urinary Tract Infection

In addition to drinking lots of water and cranberry juice, baking soda not only helps to relieve the discomfort of a urinary tract infection, it can actually help treat the condition by reducing acid in the urine. This is also achieved by drinking a concoction of baking soda and water, as noted above.

Possible Cancer Prevention and Support For Those With Cancer

Research has found that a highly acidic environment can stimulate invasive tumor growth in primary as well as metastatic cancer types. Consuming baking soda has been shown to increase the pH of tumors and slow the formation of spontaneous metastases in mice with breast cancer. It's also been found to decrease the rate of lymph node involvement and reduce the occurrence that the cancer would spread to the liver. It does this without affecting the pH balance of healthy blood and tissues. When one has a pH imbalance, potentially harmful organisms can flourish, ultimately damaging organs and tissues, as well as compromising the immune system.

In addition to helping prevent the development of cancer, a baking soda/water tonic (dissolve one to two teaspoons in a glass of filtered water) consumed once each day can provide both immune and nutritional support for those with the disease. The experts note the baking soda may also enhance the effects of conventional chemotherapy treatment. Tumor acidosis promotes chemoresistance with specific chemotherapy treatments, including paclitaxel and doxorubicin.

Cambridge Research Institute at the University of Cambridge Professor Kevin Brindle noted:

"This technique could be used as a highly-sensitive early warning system for the signs of cancer. By exploiting the body's natural pH balancing system, we have found a potentially safe way of measuring pH to see what's going on inside patients. MRIs can pick up on the abnormal pH levels found in cancer and it is possible that this could be used to pinpoint where the disease is present and when it is responding to treatment."

Preventing and Relieving Painful Kidney Stones

Baking soda makes the urine less acidic, which in turn makes uric acid kidney stone formation less likely, according to University of Michigan Health. You can use it as part of a potent recipe to internally cleanse the kidneys and remove the acid, alkalizing the body quickly. To do so, mix up 2 tablespoons of apple cider vinegar with a 1/2 teaspoon of baking soda in an 8 to 12-ounce glass of water. Drink this three times each day and it will help to decrease stone formation while removing material that causes kidney stones.

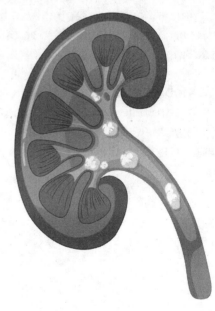

Treating Kidney Disease

A 2009 study published in the *Journal of the American Society of Nephrology* led researchers from the Department of Renal Medicine and Transplantation, at the William Harvey Research Institute Barts, and the London NHS Trust in London to summarize:

"A daily dose of baking soda could help patients with chronic kidney disease avoid having to undergo dialysis." It stated that their research showed sodium bicarbonate can dramatically slow the progress of the condition. Giving patients a small daily dose of sodium bicarbonate over a year, had only two-thirds of the decline in kidney function experienced by people given usual care.

"This cheap and simple strategy has the potential of translating into significant economic, quality of life and clinical outcome benefits," researcher Dr. Magdi Yaqoob of Royal London Hospital in the U.K., said in a news release.

Yaqoob also noted that chronic kidney disease patients with low bicarbonate levels can develop other problems, adding that a "simple remedy like sodium bicarbonate (baking soda), when used appropriately, can be very effective."

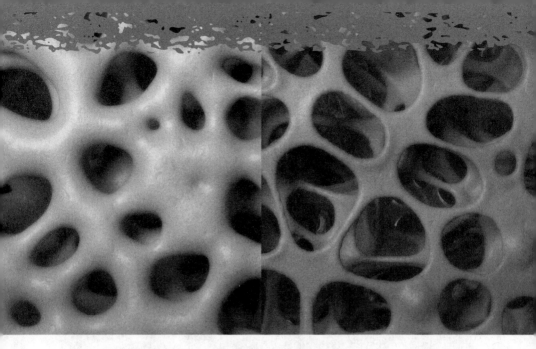

Reduce the Risk of Osteoporosis

As most people's diets are too acidic, it can lead to a loss of bone mineral density, and possibly the devastating bone disease known as osteoporosis. The consequences of this disease can affect someone for life. If it isn't prevented in the early stages, or is left untreated, it can progress without one knowing, until a bone breaks. Although the hips, wrists and spine are the most common places for an osteoporosis-related bone fracture, almost any bone can be susceptible. Drinking the mixture of one to two teaspoons of baking soda in a glass of water daily can lower your risk of developing this condition.

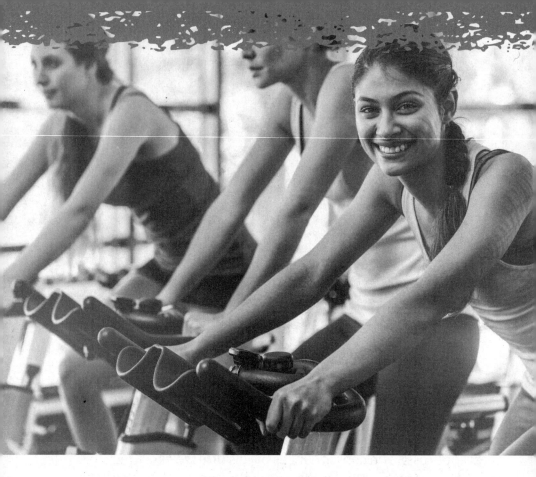

Enhance Workouts

Baking soda may enhance the effects of your workouts to help you achieve your goals faster. Research published in the European Journal of Applied Physiology in 2013 showed that consuming baking soda an hour before a lower-body strength-training session helped participants complete more repetitions with fewer signs of muscular fatigue as compared to those provided with a placebo.

That's because when you exercise near or at your maximum intensity, your muscles start to make more lactic acid. When that substance can't be processed as quickly as its produced, you'll start to feel the "burn," causing you to slow down or stop altogether. Lactic acid buildup creates acidity in the muscles, but by taking baking soda prior to the workout, it helps to buffer the acidity so that you'll be able to work out longer and even harder before having to stop.

Ultimately, if you do indeed work out longer and harder, you'll burn more calories which can aid weight loss efforts.

If you're a runner, a study from the School of Science and the Environment, Coventry University, Coventry, United Kingdom has suggested that consuming baking soda regularly may also improve sprint performance. Distance runners have long engaged in something referred to as "soda doping," which refers to taking baking soda capsules before races to enhance sprint performance, a practice believed to work similarly to carbohydrate loading.

Treating Hyperkalemia

Hyperkalemia is the medical term describing a level of potassium in your blood that's higher than normal. Potassium is critical to the function of nerve and muscle cells, including those in your heart. A normal blood potassium level is 3.6 to 5.2 millimoles per liter. If it's higher than 6.0 mmol/L, it can be dangerous and usually requires immediate treatment. This can be caused due to injury, surgery, acidosis and other conditions. Fortunately, baking soda can help with this as well, depending on the specific condition. It can be used to treat hyperkalemia that is caused primarily due to acidosis or increased levels of acidity.

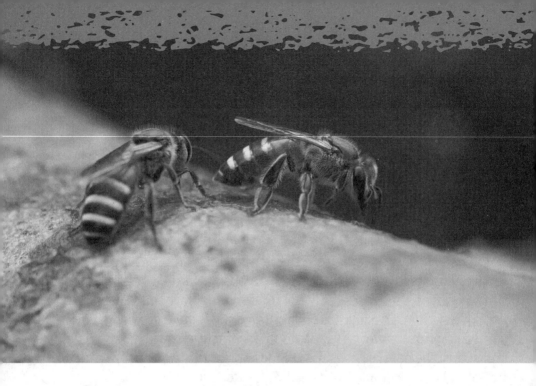

Decreasing the Pain and Swelling of a Bee or Wasp Sting

If you're stung by a bee or a wasp, the affected area often swells, and it can be very painful. Baking soda can help reduce the swelling as well as the pain caused by an insect sting. Use a solution with a high ratio of baking soda to water, at least 3:1, as a thick paste and apply it to the sting. Cover it with a bandage and re-apply as needed.

Minimize Metabolic Acidosis

Baking soda can help minimize the risk of metabolic acidosis that can occur in a number of health conditions such as cardiovascular disorders, diabetes and renal tubular acidosis. For this purpose, aim to drink a glass of water combined with a teaspoon or two of baking soda daily.

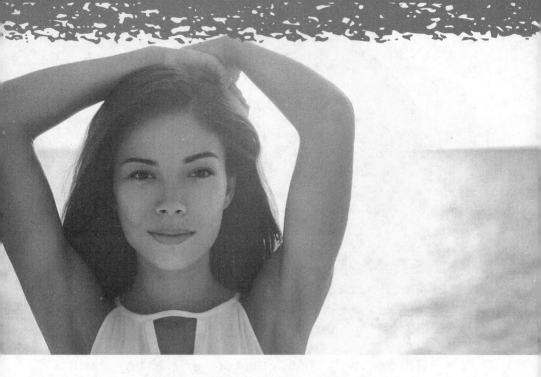

Baking Soda For Beauty

Many of us think about the food we put into our bodies, but we don't think much about the beauty products we use. Most are loaded with all sorts of chemicals, and unlike food, things like cosmetics, shampoos and creams aren't filtered through the digestive system, which means there's no way for potential toxins to be eliminated.

According to a survey by the Environmental Working Group, the average woman uses 12 products containing 168 different ingredients daily, while men use an average of six products with 85 unique ingredients each day. This essentially means that we are rubbing, lathering and bathing ourselves with dozens of chemicals every single day. And, nearly all potential toxins can penetrate the skin and get into the bloodstream. In fact, some are ingested directly from our lips or hands.

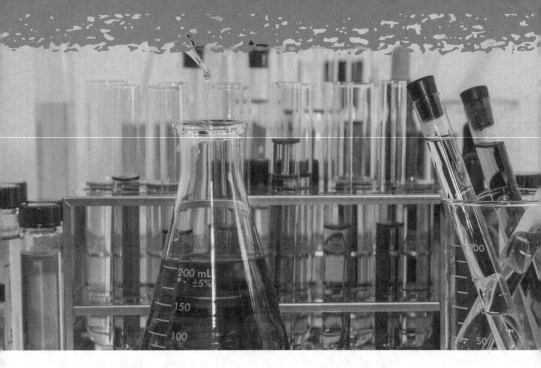

The EWG also reports that one in eight of the 82,000 ingredients in personal care products are industrial chemicals. That includes pesticides, carcinogens, hormone disruptors and reproductive toxins. Over a third of those products contain at least one ingredient that's been associated with cancer. But frighteningly, less than 20 percent of the chemicals in these types of products have been tested for safety. That's because the Food and Drug Administration (FDA) does not limit or regulate the use of chemicals in personal care products, or even require that all of the ingredients be listed on the label.

Here's just one example: deodorant. Around 95 percent of Americans use deodorant in an attempt to adhere to social norms and smell fresher, but in the process they're frequently subjecting themselves to a host of negative side effects due to all of those chemicals and other toxic ingredients they contain. One of those offending compounds in conventional deodorant is the antibacterial agent called triclosan.

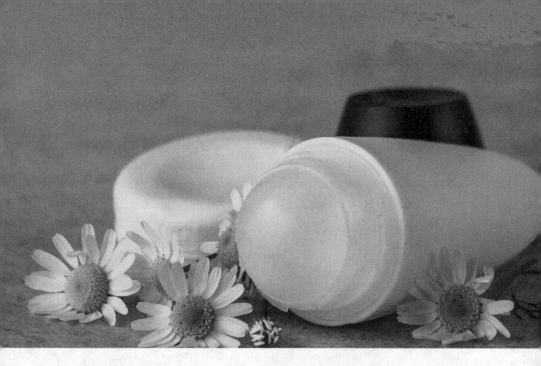

Triclosan is commonly found in deodorants, as well as some soaps and other personal care items, but it's been flagged as a serious risk to both humans and the environment. Research has found that triclosan can alter hormone regulation, and it also contributes to the worldwide problem of antibiotic resistant bacteria. It's also been shown in studies to have a connection to weight gain, the inflammatory response, allergies and thyroid dysfunction. Not only that, but the aluminum compounds that are typically in store-bought deodorants are known to block sweat ducts and mimic estrogen which can promote the growth of breast cancer cells. Those conventional deodorants usually contain parabens too, which are also linked to breast cancer.

The list goes on and on. When University of California, Berkeley researchers tested 32 lipsticks and lip glosses that are found in drugstores and department stores across the U.S., ranging in price from $5 to $24, they found concerning levels of nine heavy metals, including lead, cadmium, chromium, aluminum and five others. Conventional creams often contain alkyloamides, which are used as emulsifiers, emollients and thickening agents, like DEA, TEA or MEA.

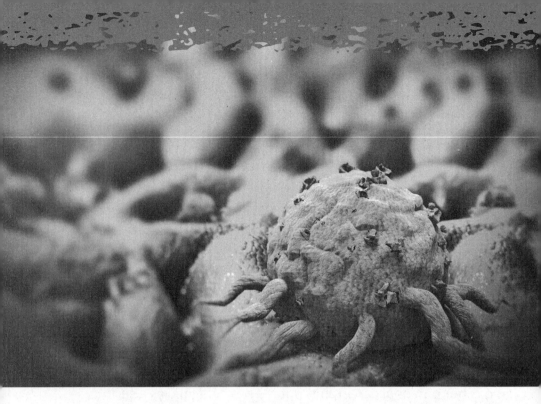

Although they aren't considered toxic themselves, they can become contaminated with nitrosamines, compounds that are considered cancer-causing.

If that isn't enough to make you think about switching up your beauty regimen, we're not sure what will. Of course, we're not recommending you give it up altogether, rather to consider using natural alternatives, like baking soda, something just about everyone already has in their kitchen cabinets.

Sodium bicarbonate, or baking soda, is a practically miraculous product — it's cheap, non-toxic and it can be used in many effective beauty product recipes, not to mention its uses for household cleaning and cooking.

Now is the time to stock up, as you'll be able to replace many of those expensive chemical-filled products by taking advantage of that famous white stuff in the little orange box.

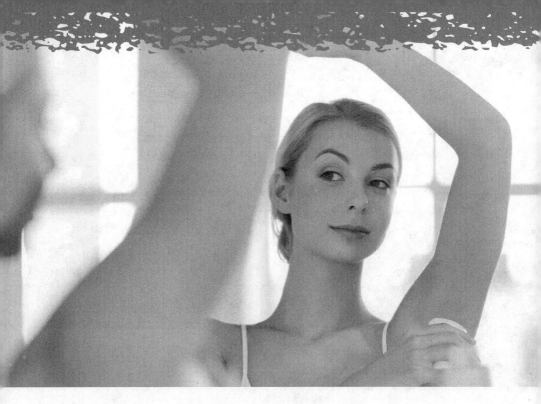

Deodorant

Speaking of deodorant, you can actually use baking soda to create your own natural product to kill body odor. You can simply mix four tablespoons of sodium bicarbonate with five to ten drops of your favorite essential oil to add a pleasant scent, and apply the mixture to your underarms. Also, try this highly effective recipe.

Ingredients

- 1/4 cup baking soda
- 1/4 cup cornstarch
- 6 tbsp coconut oil, melted
- 10 drops essential oil as desired (optional)

Instructions

1. Mix all ingredients well.
2. Use a cotton pad or tissue to apply to your underarms.

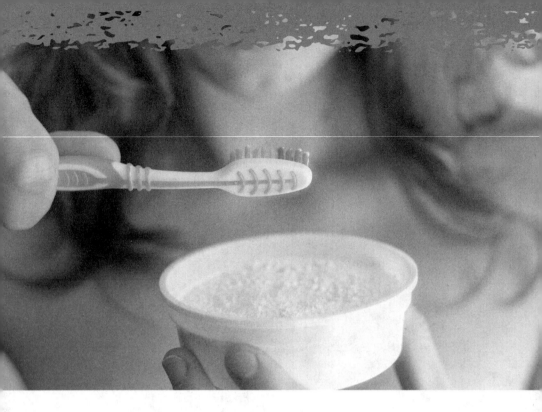

Toothpaste and Whitener

Using baking soda as an ingredient in toothpaste is a great way to keep teeth shiny and white. Simply mix a little into coconut oil to create a paste and then add a drop of peppermint essential oil. You can get them extra white by combining a teaspoon of baking soda with one fresh, mashed strawberry. Apply the mixture to your teeth and leave it on as long as you can while resisting the urge to swallow, and then rinse.

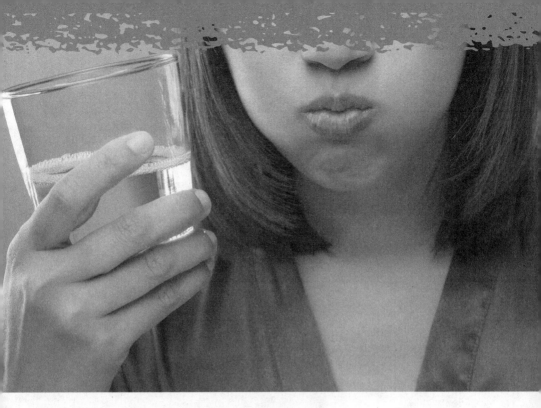

Mouthwash

For a cheap, natural mouthwash without toxins, add a half-teaspoon of baking soda to about four ounces of warm water, and use it to gargle. It's an instant fix for even the worst bad breath. If you have dry mouth, combine a cup of warm water, one-eighth teaspoon of sea salt and one-quarter teaspoon baking soda. Swish small sips of it in your mouth and then rinse with plain water.

These baking soda recipes work because sodium carbonate serves to neutralize the odors in your mouth, instead of simply covering them up. It has an alkaline pH that balances against the acids that are produced by bacteria in your mouth, especially from acidic drinks like soda and coffee.

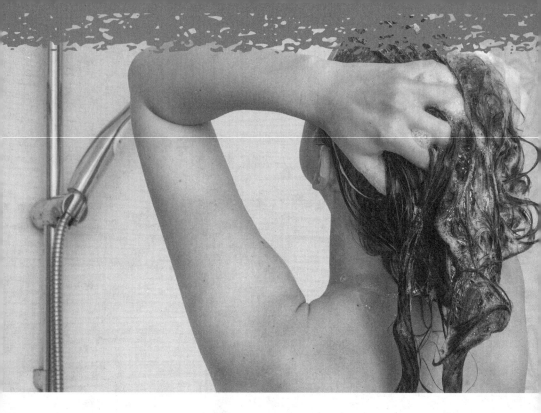

Shampoo

Is there anything baking soda can't do? It even works wonders as a shampoo. It helps to remove styling product buildup which results in healthier, more manageable hair. All you have to do to use it is wet your hair and then sprinkle about a tablespoon onto your scalp. Massage it gently into your roots and then rinse just like you would with traditional shampoo.

By following this process with an apple cider vinegar rinse, it will help to balance the alkalinity of baking soda, further remove buildup and residue, and close the hair cuticles. Pour about a half cup of apple cider vinegar over your hair after the baking soda shampoo treatment and then rinse once again.

This effective technique is sometimes referred to as the "no-poo" method, and many swear by it to maintain their beautiful, long locks.

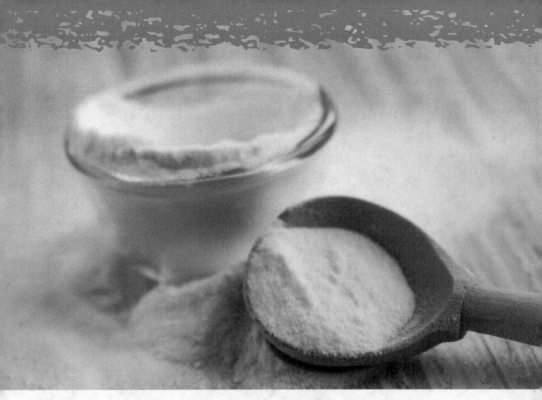

Dry Shampoo

No time to shower but hair is in need of refreshing? Instead, sprinkle a little baking soda across the roots of your hair and tossle it around a bit to work it in. Instantly, you'll have refreshed, deodorized, rejuvenated hair.

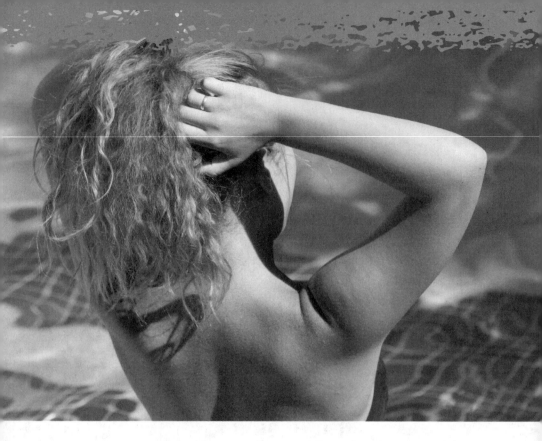

Get Rid of Chlorine Hair

If you're a swimmer, you know the kind of damage chlorine can do to your hair. That stuff used to keep harmful bacteria out of the pool water can also strip your hair of its natural oils, leaving it dry and brittle. To remove it, try the Kool-Aid trick, which includes baking soda, of course. It will also work to get out the brassiness and mineral buildup. Simply mix a little lemonade Kool-Aid powder with a dollop of dish soap and a bit of baking soda. Follow that up with a good conditioner to moisturize.

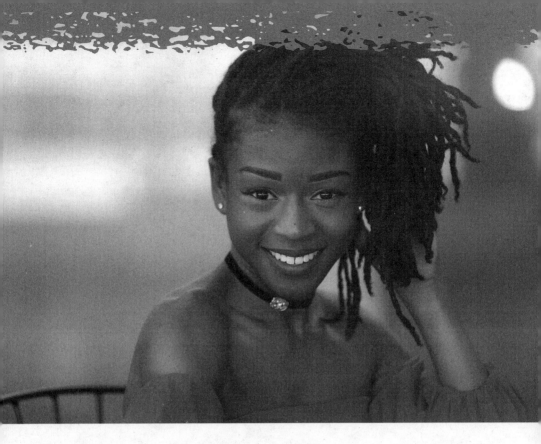

Wash Dreadlocks

Dreadlocks can be challenging to maintain, but you can use baking soda to keep them clean and odor-free. Combine a three-quarter cup baking soda with a gallon of water. Then add two tablespoons sea salt, two tablespoons lemon juice and about 20 drops of lavender essential oil. Pour this over your head and let your hair soak it up for ten to 15 minutes. Rinse well.

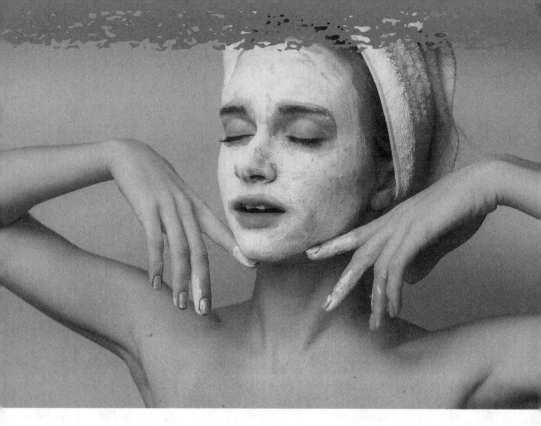

Acne Mask

You can zap those frustrating zits by making a mask using baking soda that's designed to fight acne. Just mix up equal amounts of honey and baking soda, and then apply it as a spot treatment. Allow the mixture to sit for about 15 minutes and then rinse thoroughly.

If you have stubborn blackheads, combine a tablespoon of sodium bicarbonate with a quarter-cup of milk. Rub the paste into affected areas, using it like an exfoliating scrub. After letting it sit for a few minutes, rinse as normal.

Beautify Your Feet

Cracked, dry heels are common during a cold, harsh winter, but other things can cause that problem too, including dehydration if you aren't drinking enough water, failing to moisturize your feet, using harsh soaps or chemical-filled products on them, or taking particularly hot showers or baths. Fortunately, this unsightly and often painful problem can be easily fixed by using a little baking soda. The baking soda helps to exfoliate the skin to make it nice and smooth, while its deodorizing properties work to remove foot odor, and it will also aid in cleaning the bottoms of your feet to prevent any cracks from becoming infected.

Ingredients

- A bathtub, container or bucket
- Baking soda
- Water
- Pumice stone
- Coconut oil
- Lavender essential oil
- Socks

Instructions

1. Add about three tablespoons of baking soda to a container or bucket that's filled with water, or five tablespoons of baking soda to your partially-filled bathtub.

2. Soak your feet for about 20 minutes. Afterwards, use the pumice stone to scrub your heels until smooth — avoid scrubbing to hard to prevent damaging the skin.

3. Add a couple drops of lavender essential oil to coconut oil, making enough to rub into the bottoms of both feet. Massage in the mixture, concentrating on the heels.

4. Put the socks on to help trap the moisture in. Repeat the process three times a week until your feet have healed, and then once a week after that to keep them that way.

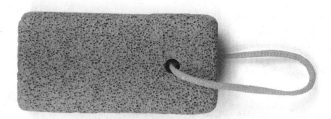

If you have tough calluses you want to soften, baking soda can help with that too. Just add a tablespoon to a basin of warm water along with a few drops of lavender essential oil. Enjoy a nice, long, relaxing soak and then scrub those calluses away using a combination of three parts baking soda, one part water and one part brown sugar.

Keep Your Combs and Brushes Clean

If your combs or brushes aren't kept clean, that residue, the oils, dead skin cells and so on will colonize the brush, and they can provide the ideal environment for yeast and bacteria to reside. This is bad for your hair and it can start to smell bad, too. Cleaning your hair brushes and combs once a week will keep them from building up all of that gunk, and allow them to do their job, which is to grip the hair and smooth out the cuticle.

Baking soda is great for this purpose, naturally removing all of that residue, build up and oils. All you have to do is soak your brushes in a solution of one cup water and a teaspoon of baking soda. Afterwards, rinse and dry thoroughly. You can use a blow dryer to get them dry faster.

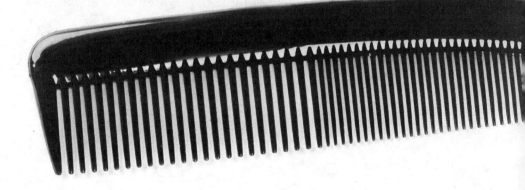

Gently Cleaning Extra-Dirty Hands

If your hands are really dirty after digging in your garden, or some other task, don't use a harsh soap as it can irritate the skin on your hands and lead to painful cracking or itching. Instead, gently wash your hands using a paste made up of one part water to three parts baking soda. It will leave your hands clean and super soft.

Enhance a Manicure

If you want a salon-type manicure at home, take advantage of that box of baking soda. Use a small nail brush, dip it into some baking soda, and then gently scrub with it. Make sure to get underneath your nails and around your cuticles until they're all clean. Next, make a paste using three parts baking soda to one part water. Gently rub the paste in a circular motion over your hands and fingers to exfoliate and smooth the skin. Afterwards, rinse with warm water, moisturize and then apply your nail polish as usual.

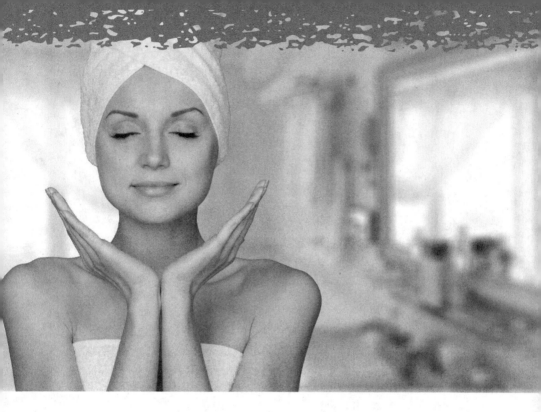

Brighten Your Complexion

To brighten a dull complexion, combine a tablespoon of lemon juice, a few drops of extra-virgin olive oil and enough baking soda to make a paste. After washing your skin as usual, apply this paste all over your face, avoiding the eye area. Allow it to sit for about ten minutes and then rinse with cool water. It will leave your face brighter, while softening and hydrating your skin.

Heal a Rash

Baking soda combined with coconut oil provides soothing anti-inflammatory and antibacterial properties, and also works wonders on skin rashes. Simply mix coconut oil and baking soda until you've achieved the consistency of a paste. Apply the paste to the affected area and allow it to remain for five minutes before rinsing off with cool water. Repeat daily until the rash has healed.

Artificial Tan Remover

Most of us have probably attempted to self-tan, wishing for that beautiful summer bronzed look only to end up with unsightly streaks, or, perhaps even worse, orange glowing skin. Not exactly what you hoped to achieve, right? If that happens again, you'll know what to do. There's no reason to hide until it eventually fades away. Instead, make a body exfoliator that will get rid of it in minutes. Just combine one part water to three parts baking soda, apply it to that unsightly "tan," and gently scrub it away.

Soothe Razor Burn

No one wants stray hairs sticking out of their bathing suit, but razor burn around the bikini line is oh-so-painful, not to mention unsightly — almost as bad as the hairs that were there in the first place! Fortunately, you can soothe that sensitive skin using a solution of one cup water and one tablespoon of baking soda. Apply this paste to your skin and allow it to dry, typically about five minutes. Once it's completely dry, you can rinse it off with cool water.

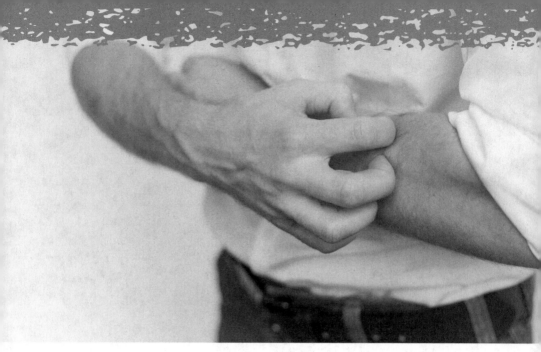

Relieve Itchy Skin

The cold winter months can leave your skin feeling rather uncomfortable, dry and itchy. While a hot bath feels good, it makes that dry skin problem even worse. Instead, add a half-cup of baking soda to warm water, along with about ten drops of vetiver essential oil. Distilled from the roots of the vetiver plant, this oil helps to bring moisture to dry skin and relief to that itch. In fact, in India they call it the oil of tranquility, and it will surely help to bring peace of mind when that uncomfortable feeling dissipates. Enjoy a nice soak and when you step out of the bath, your skin will feel soft and smooth. Applying coconut, olive or almond oil afterwards is optional for extra moisture.

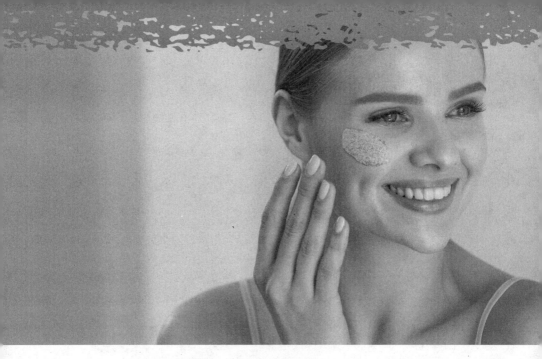

Exfoliate Your Face For a Beautiful, Glowing Look

To get rid of dead skin cells and leave your face with a beautiful, glowing look, use baking soda as an exfoliator. You can simply combine a tablespoon of baking soda with a little water to make a paste, or add the liquid from inside a vitamin E pill for extra benefits. Adding a drop or two of lavender essential oil will help moisturize and prevent breakouts.

Simply mix all of the ingredients together in a small bowl to create a paste — it shouldn't be too runny or too thick. Wash your face as you normally would, leaving it a bit damp, and then apply the paste. Gently rub it in using small circular motions, avoiding the eye area while covering your cheeks, forehead, chin and lips. Leave the paste on for a few minutes and then rinse with cool water, making sure to remove all granules. Gently pat your face dry and follow with a moisturizer — coconut oil is ideal.

Fade Dark Spots, Moles and Freckles

If you have dark spots, moles or freckles on your skin, you can lighten them so they aren't as noticeable by using this baking soda recipe. It's effective because using baking soda, when combined with other ingredients, helps to form a caustic solution that helps dehydrate and bleach dark areas on the skin.

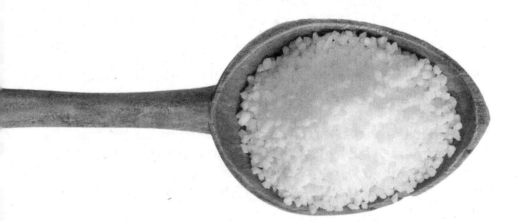

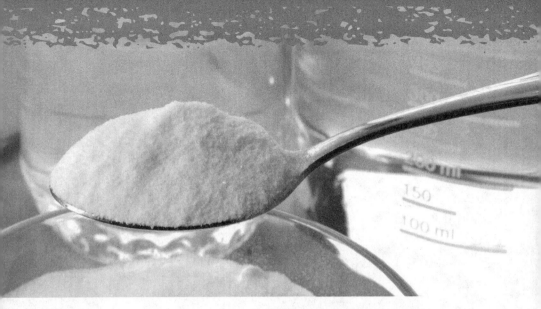

Ingredients

- 1 cup baking soda
- 1 cup hydrogen peroxide (3% solution)
- 1 cup Epsom salt
- 1/4 cup boiling water
- 1/4 cup white vinegar
- Bottle for storage

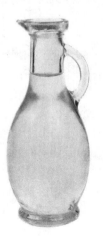

Instructions

1. Combine the baking soda, Epsom salt and hydrogen peroxide.

2. Add boiling water to the mixture and combine thoroughly.

3. Add in white vinegar, stir again to combine and then add the entire solution to the storage bottle.

4. Apply the solution to freckles, moles, dark spots, etc., allowing it to remain for about 20 minutes.

5. Rinse well.

6. Follow this process twice each day until you achieve the results you're looking for.

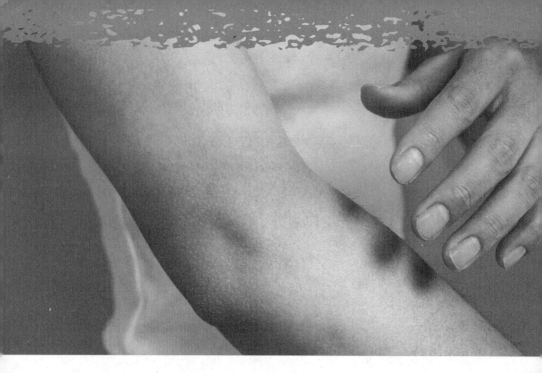

Soothe a Sunburn

If your skin is red and painful after spending too much time in the sun, you'll be glad to know that baking soda can easily help you put together an effective home remedy that you can use to feel better. While it won't cure your sunburn (only time will do that), it should ease the pain and stinging to make it easier for you to live with the redness while your skin heals.

There are two ways to use baking soda for this purpose. First, you can simply add it to your bath and enjoy a soothing soak. Fill up your bathtub with water that's cool to the touch, and while it's filling, add a cup of baking soda. Relax in the tub for a while and you'll soon notice your skin starting to feel better. Another option is to mix baking soda and water into a paste to apply to your sunburn for relief. Start with a half-cup of baking soda in a bowl, adding cool water until the mixture is thin enough to spread onto your sunburned skin. Apply this paste onto sunburned areas, and allow it to remain for 15 to 20 minutes before rinsing off with cool water.

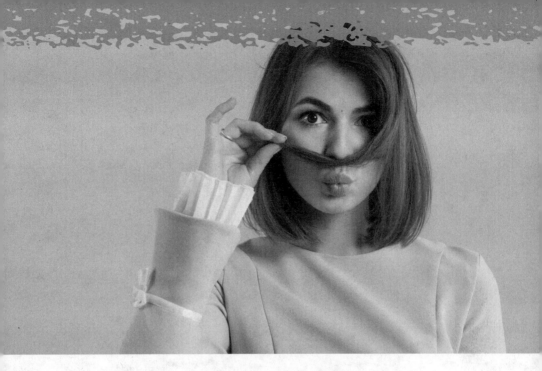

Remove Facial Hair

Many women have facial hair they'd like to get rid of, and baking soda can even help with this problem too. Combine a tablespoon of baking soda with about two cups of boiling water. Allow the solution to cool and then soak a piece of cotton in it. Drain the cotton so it isn't dripping, and then secure it to the area you'd like to remove hair with a bandage, like a Band-Aid. If you have more than one area, repeat the process on those areas too. Leave the bandages on overnight, and then in the morning remove them. The solution will work to dehydrate hair follicles and damage them, which causes the hair to fall out. Note, as this can cause skin irritation in some people, you may want to use on only a small area first.

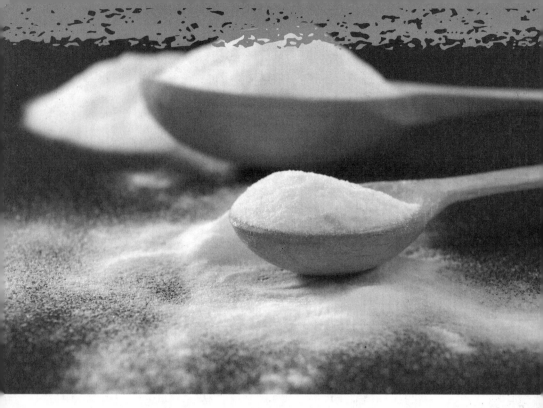

Stock Up

Now you can see why it's imperative to keep baking soda in your kitchen, garden shed and even your medicine cabinet, right? Stock up when it goes on sale and be sure to never underestimate its power to clean, refresh and remedy!